Intergenerational Arts in the Nursing Home

Intergenerational Arts in the Nursing Home

A Handbook

PATCH CLARK

GREENWOOD PRESS
New York • Westport, Connecticut • London

Library of Congress Cataloging-in-Publication Data

Clark, Patch.
    Intergenerational arts in the nursing home : a handbook / Patch
Clark.
        p. cm.
        Includes bibliographical references and index.
        ISBN 0-313-25965-8 (alk. paper)
        1. Arts and the aged—United States.   2. Nursing homes—United
States—Recreational activities.   I. Title.
    NX180.A35C5   1991
    362.1'6—dc20   91-138

British Library Cataloguing in Publication Data is available.

Library of Congress Catalog Card Number: 91-138
ISBN: 0-313-25965-8

First published in 1991

Greenwood Press, 88 Post Road West, Westport, CT   06881
An imprint of Greenwood Publishing Group, Inc.

Printed in the United States of America

The paper used in this book complies with the
Permanent Paper Standard issued by the National
Information Standards Organization (Z39.48-1984).

10 9 8 7 6 5 4 3 2 1

Copyright Acknowledgments

Grateful acknowledgment is given for permission to use excerpts from the following:

M. Sorgman, M. Sorenson, and M. Johnston, "What Sounds Do I Make When I'm Old?" from *Social Education* 43 (1979). Used by permission of the National Council for the Social Studies.

Excerpts from "Miss Leonora When Last Seen" from *The Collected Stories* by Peter Taylor. Copyright © 1960, 1969 by Peter Taylor. Renewal copyright © 1988 by Peter Taylor. Reprinted by permission of Farrar, Straus and Giroux, Inc.

M. Naumburg, "Spontaneous Art in Education and Psychotherapy," in *Art Therapy in Theory and Practice,* 2nd ed., edited by E. Ulman and P. Dachinger, copyright © 1977. By permission of Random House.

M. Centron, B. Soriano, and M. Gale, *Schools of the Future: How American Business Can Cooperate to Save Our Schools,* copyright © 1985. By permission of the publisher, McGraw-Hill, Inc.

James Halpern, *Helping Your Aging Parents,* copyright © 1987. Published by Fawcett Press and reproduced by permission of McGraw-Hill, Inc.

Michael Kirby, "Introduction," originally published in *The Drama Review* 20, no. 1 (1976). Used by permission of the MIT Press.

R. Bausell, A. Rooney, C. Inlander, *How to Evaluate and Select a Nursing Home*, copyright © 1988, by Addison-Wesley Publishing Co., Inc., Reading, Massachusetts. Reprinted with permission of the publisher.

M. Dellmann-Jenkins, D. Lambert, D. Fruit, and T. Dinero, "Old and Young Together: Effect of an Educational Program on Preschoolers' Attitudes Toward Older People," *Childhood Education* 62 (1986). Reprinted by permission of M. Dellmann-Jenkins and the Association for Childhood Education International, 11141 Georgia Avenue, Suite 200, Wheaton, MD. Copyright © 1986 by the Association.

B. Davis, "Drama: A Tool for Nutrition Education with Older Adults," *Journal of Nutrition Education* 15 (1983): 5. Copyright © Society of Nutritional Education.

D. Zahler and K. A. Zahler, *Test Your Cultural Literacy,* copyright © 1988. Reprinted by permission of the publisher, ARCO, Simon & Schuster, Inc., New York, NY 10023.

Excerpt from *The Living Theatre* by Elmer Rice. Copyright © 1959 by Elmer Rice. Reprinted by permission of HarperCollins Publishers.

Barbara Cooney, *Miss Rumphius,* copyright © 1982 by Barbara Cooney Porter. Reprinted by permission of Penguin Books USA Inc.

Gay and Kathlyn Hendricks, *The Moving Center,* copyright © 1983. Reprinted by permission of the publisher, Prentice-Hall/A division of Simon & Schuster, Inc., New York, NY 10023.

R. Laban and F. C. Lawrence, *Effort: Economy in Body Movement,* copyright © 1974. Reprinted by permission of Pitman Publishing.

C. Ventura-Merkel and L. Lidoff, *Community Planning for Intergenerational Programming,* © and reprinted with permission of The National Council on the Aging, 600 Maryland Avenue SW, West Wing 100, Washington, DC 22024.

Every reasonable effort has been made to trace the owners of copyright materials in this book, but in some instances this has proven impossible. The author and publisher will be glad to receive information leading to more complete acknowledgments in subsequent printings of the book and in the meantime extend their apologies for any omissions.

TO
FRANK, BARBARA, GINNY, RON, ROB,
AND
MY PARENTS

Contents

Preface

It is interesting to note that in today's modern society we look to the aged for wisdom. Or do we? This is one of the questions posed over and over again as we look for stability in an ever-changing world. Geographical boundaries transpose, political power reverses, companies merge and dissolve, scientific discoveries proliferate and in the midst of all this we try to maintain some sense of security. But does change guarantee success or improvement? Are we equipped to meet the challenge of the twenty-first century as parents, workers, and educators, as people uncertain of outcomes? It has been the experience of mankind to look to someone more knowledgeable, more experienced, when searching for a solution to a problem. In past decades the persons who held such knowledge were the elders of our society.

Throughout the history of America there have been waves of efforts, both social and political, to assist the elderly in maintaining their respected position in our society. Yet, at some point, the positive public image of aging began to diminish. Instead of becoming an invaluable source of knowledge and wisdom, the elderly were perceived as a burden upon society. They were seen as being at a place in the life-span where nobody wanted to go or be. Their presence affirmed that one's life does indeed eventually end. However, for many elderly persons, life begins during these later years.

Enter the youth of America, who have been seen both as a blessing and, sadly enough, as a hindrance. Sometimes their public image suffers as much as does that of the elderly. Picture, for a moment, a young man helping an old woman across the street. The old woman gently pats the young man on the head as they reach the curb. She meekly offers him a quarter, but he shakes his head, indicating that his good deed has come from the heart. They go on their respective ways, smiling. It is an image that we smile at; yet if we say "youth" or "elderly" in separate breaths, the positive vision may become questionable, if not cloudy.

During the early seventies there was a surge of interest in the arts and the elderly. Within the context of this book we shall begin to examine some of the programs that have quietly and steadily grown and flourished. From these programs came other programs, born in the eighties. As we enter the nineties, however, cutbacks in federal and state government spending, make their future questionable. It has become necessary to look for other ways to support, maintain, and develop valuable programs.

The elderly are not the only ones faced with unfortunate circumstances. The youth in our educational systems are dangerously faced with a less-than-adequate education to meet the demands of the nineties. As funding is cut, more and more youngsters cannot possibly be prepared with the skills needed to take us into the twenty-first century.

Enter the parents, who have every right to be frightened about their children's preparation for the future. Their fear is justified not because knowledge, work, and devotion are lacking in educators, but because the necessary funding is lacking to maintain quality education.

The last players to enter this stage of events are the businesses. While some are enjoying growth and stability, others are concerned about the quality of work and the educational skills of their workers and about the long-term projections of their companies.

The director of this life-show becomes the moving force that brings all of the elements together. The children, the parents, the elderly, the educators, and the businessmen and businesswomen must become the focused and creative directors in producing the next chapter in the successful life performance of humanity. Through the collaborative effort of these groups we will develop a newly defined intergenerational base group that will have a greater impact upon society than could any single group.

It is exciting to discover such exemplary programs as the Arts Mentor Program, a program of the National Council on the Aging; the Performing Tree, "a community-based, private, non-profit educational organization dedicated to children and their need for dance, music, theatre, and the literary and visual arts as essential elements in their basic education," which also implements the program Senior Folk Artists in the Classroom; and the Palmcrest House in Long Beach, California, which offers such special celebrations as "A Fantasy Island Adventure" and art exhibits at the Senior Eye Gallery. These three programs and a multitude of other excellent projects attest to the shared interests among the generations in the visual and performing arts.

It is time for a renewed sense of history to be shared by those involved in the making of history. If we are to look to the past for advice or wisdom, we must also look to the future for successful survival. As we move from individual efforts into an era of shared responsibility, it will become more and more evident that the ideas, knowledge, and experiences of all ages are needed in order to meet the demands of the twenty-first century.

There is something to be said for the concern over the rise of violence in our nation and the breakdown of the family unit. As more and more families must have two parents at work, children are forced to look towards a system of "extended" family for guidance, assistance with learning, and even basic social skills. Where before in our history we have had guiding mentors who have been able to say, "Now, when everybody in the family has to go off to work, this is how we can maintain some unity, some security, some focus"? For the most part, we are a collection of generations who have only learned about the breakdown of the family unit through war, divorce, and the industrial revolution which brought about an entire economic-societal change. We are now on the verge of learning how to cope with the results. What have we learned?

Educators say we have learned that parents are vitally important to the success of their child's educational career. Parents say that their families are becoming ever increasingly important to them, especially in a two-career family. The elderly say that life is still important to them and that they might be able to help out...if only someone will take heed.

Turning points in literature almost always present the highest point of action, deliberation, or contemplation. We are at a turning point in the history of mankind, whereby families can be reunited, reinvented, renewed, or redesigned. It is, afterall, through the old-fashioned family values of helping one another, listening to one another, and responding to one another that nations, cultures, and civilizations exist and thrive. The difference in the family structure, however, exists in the demographic, economic, and geographic changes since the Industrial Revolution. Now, the child must learn from perhaps someone else's grandfather or grandmother, but the lessons are still as valuable, still as urgent, and still as caring as if we were all still living under the same roof.

Through the chapters of this book we will investigate, discover, and contemplate previous programs, existing programs, and ideas for future programs that will create a new sense of family. The honorable living resources in our nursing homes will, we hope, become the surrogate stabilizers of a working society and pass on valuable lessons of living, hope, and discovery as we proceed into the twenty-first century. The young person and the old woman will again cross the street together, but perhaps, sometime in the near future, they will both be headed in the same direction.

Intergenerational Arts in the Nursing Home

1
Developing a New Sense
of Culture

THE INTERGENERATIONAL CIVILIZATION

In his book *Cultural Literacy: What Every American Needs To Know,* E.D. Hirsch states,"In early grades our children were taught texts with cultural content rather than 'developmental' texts that develop abstract skills...." He goes on to suggest that,"our children's lack of intergenerational information is a serious problem for the nation" (1987, p.7). Although the 1960s brought to the nation a fight for equality, the 1970s brought, through specialization, a separatist phenomenon to the generations. Even among public schools the movement was away from housing successive generations in the same building. Although a surge of development in long-term health care facilities and a subsequent quest for excellence are beginning to meet the needs of our ever-growing elderly population, the move away from the mainstream of community life has taken its toll on the relationship between our youth and our society. Our youth are being deprived of an important facet of their education-that of learning from their elders. The consequences reach beyond educational dimensions: that the youth also are failing to learn about and cope with their own aging process.

In correcting a societal deficit, the first step is to seek the cause of the problem. It is unfair to blame the health care institutions, for they are doing everything in their power to improve the quality of life. Does the blame lie with the educational system? They, too, are trying to keep up with the soaring costs and demands of educating young people. Should we then go back and study the Industrial Age and the separation of families carried through to the Information Age of the 1980s? The development of machines has indeed brought peoples closer on a global level, yet what has it done to the "old-fashioned" family unit? One argument is that, because of the rapid expansion in telecommunications, families may communicate in spite of the miles that may separate them. However, communicating by a telephone call once a week, monthly, or only on holidays is quite different from growing up in the company of an elderly person and maturing as that person ages naturally.

The early learning experiences of children, whether through the mass media, books, or contact with older people, help to form important visual images that may then lead to either positive or negative understanding of other human beings. "By a logical extension, the views which the children hold today of the aged might be expected to have a strong influence upon their adult reactions to the aged, and also to color their self-concept when they themselves are elderly" (T. Hickey, L. Hickey, and R. Kalish, 1968, p. 227). Judith Powell and George Arquitt further support this notion, saying, "the way in which older adults are treated in our society is determined, in part, by the way younger generations perceive them. Older people are disappearing from children's lives, and many young people are growing up with little or no opportunity to have meaningful relationships with the elderly" (p.421, 1978). The sound of a mother's or, more recently, the father's voice as he or she reads to a baby or young child begins the process of life's investigation. Opinions are formed early and broken late.

Because of the migration of younger generations away from the parental home, families are now separated, sometimes by continents. For the most part children no longer grow up near grandparents. "The fragmentation of the extended family, the elimination of the neighborhood as a social entity, and the emphasis on age segregated voluntary associations have decreased the opportunity for establishing meaningful contacts between the old and young" (Powell and Arquitt, p. 421). Children's opinions are formed early by what they see on television, by what they hear, and by the people with whom they come into contact. If less-than-positive opinions are initially formed, then passage into adolescence, a time when peer pressure and glowing physical appearance take precedence, may bring about an even more negative view of the aging process.

At first, my high school students have a difficult time going to the nursing home with me because they say it is "depressing." When asked to elaborate further upon their feelings, they respond that they find the sense of helplessness and hopelessness frustrating. They repeatedly ask, "Is this the end of working so hard in school, studying, getting a job, and raising a family?" But what they don't see, until they have had an opportunity to maintain weekly contact, is the "individualism" of each resident and a new beginning in yet another stage of life. Until students experience regular contact with the elderly and become acquainted with them as human beings, rather than as a stereotypical group, they continue to harbor this negative image. Until they understand and appreciate the individual personalities and see each as a person who can still contribute thoughts and ideas to a conversation, to another person's life, to the world, they remain in the power of a negative force, unable to move toward human understanding.

For America's youth, contact with persons in long-term care facilities is vitally important to the continued strength and revitalization of the family unit. The importance of this contact is twofold. First of all, the youth of today are in need of a respite from the pressures of daily living. The external pressures of grades, finances, and friends only fuel the internal fires of the need for acceptance, the longing to succeed, and the struggle for independence. Through contact with elderly people in nursing homes, adolescents are offered a rest along the wayside from cultural, parental, and educational pressures. For the most part, those confined to nursing homes welcome visitors with whom they might converse, share, or even just sit quietly. It is an opportunity to slow down, to be completely removed from the bustling society that requires so much of a young person. This is not to say, however, that nursing homes are not busy. Quite the contrary. But there is time, quality time, to spend with visitors, especially with the younger generation. The nursing home also provides the younger generation with an opportunity to give to others. Youth are often overlooked in their ability and natural instinct to provide. Although in most public high schools, service clubs are an integral part of the learning environment, contact with the elderly in nursing homes is usually limited to the Christmas visit or other holiday celebrations. These visits are important, but why not expand this exposure, which is beneficial to all involved?

It is also important to note that the elderly may not hold the record for loneliness. "There is some evidence that older people are in fact less lonely than younger people. One survey found that the highest rate of loneliness occurred in people between the ages of 18 and 25, and some researchers believe that adolescents experience the highest rate" (Halpern, 1987, p. 92).

Another factor to consider is the rapidly changing makeup of public education. Public schools must address the increasing elderly population as well. Marvin J. Cetron, Barbara Soriano, and Margaret Gale predict that "students of the 21st century will probably include toddlers, children, youth, adults, and older citizens. A typical school district may provide learning experiences and training for students ages 3 to 21 and for adults 21 to 80-plus" (1985, p. 94). They go on to say that educational systems may also find themselves in competition for funding with health care professions. It makes sense, then, to combine the efforts of the two in a plan to improve our present and future standards for quality of life. It is entirely possible that the nursing home setting may one day become a popular retreat for all ages, a place where the gathering of minds, hearts, and talent will lead a to new examination of the values of life. The first step, however, is taken by walking into the nursing home, and unfortunately we have a negative image of the nursing home.

James Halpern advises the children of aging parents to develop an understanding of their elders that may in turn, be passed down to their children. These efforts must be expanded to advising the nation to explore, mix, and communicate:

> The elderly are your future-what everyone becomes. Helping and understanding your aging parents will enable you to get acquainted with this stage of life and be better prepared for it when you arrive there. If you show a level of affection and respect for the elderly, you teach your own children this attitude. The emotions of prejudice-ridicule, disgust, and rejection- are like most techniques, transmitted from parent to child through modeling and imitation. Ageism in our society is a reflection of a lack of self-acceptance. Many young people don't understand that there is a continuity of personality as aging progresses. The inner person does not change in the way the body does. The personality of the older person remains intact as he watches his body deteriorate. The best cure for ageism is getting to know older people....(Halpern 1987,p. 88).

Persons placed in nursing homes require a firm commitment to continued care from a responsible society. Furthermore, it is important that children continue to have the opportunity to be around the elderly and to experience either their own or "surrogate" grandparents.

It is imperative that children share positive experiences with the elderly at an early age and that the elderly continue their contact with children and young people. A vital bridge in humanity is lost when the two are separated. Age-segregation through long-term care facilities, retirement centers, and institutions of public education has become a serious problem. On the other hand, some nursing homes and public schools offer community outreach programs, serving as a "recreation" center, gathering place, and focal point of a thriving community where all ages gather to celebrate, solve problems, share ideas, and learn from one another. One approach to bringing the generations together, then, is through intergenerational programming.

VALUES OF INTERGENERATIONAL PROGRAMMING

Intergenerational programming not only helps to diffuse negative stereotypes of aging but also presents a more positive picture of long-term health care. It is indeed unfortunate that we, as a nation, harbor such negative feelings towards nursing homes. The mere mention of the term conjures up for many any number of negative thoughts. "For a variety of reasons, we generally think of nursing homes as a last resort, as a step which signals hopelessness, denoting finality, the end of growth and potential. In this view, the nursing home is a long-term, medically-oriented holding place, strictly custodial in nature, where real living and progressing ceases, and where sterility and efficiency, the 'nursing' components, take precedence over warmth and caring, the 'home' components" (Halpern 1987, p. 197).

Yet, if one has been exposed to activity programs or to high-quality nursing care in homes across the nation, one sees the opposite of this stereotypical vision.   Nurses, aides, volunteers, clergy, and visiting schoolchildren all dispel the myth of inactivity and waiting for death.   R. Barker Bausell, Michael A. Rooney and Charles B. Inlander give us a forceful thought in their *How to Evaluate and Select a Nursing Home* in stating that "a nursing home is *not* for someone who is extremely sick-a hospital is. It is also *not* a prison where people are segregated from society. It is *not* a drawn-out hospice program where people are waiting for the inevitable deterioration and death. It is, rather, a *home* for people who have difficulty caring for themselves where rehabilitation on all levels is undertaken" (1988, p. 2).

Children and young people, however, are not the only targets of misinformation and negative feelings toward nursing homes.   Many elderly people have developed the same opinions and thus, upon admittance, display embitterment, frustration, and fright.

In his discussion of minority elderly, Donald E. Gelfand states, "Perhaps the best way to conclude a discussion of services and the aged population, however, is to restress the importance of developing the positive feeling of the ethnic aged people toward service providers while avoiding the dangers of encouraging increased passivity on the part of older individuals toward changes in their lives" (Gelfand 1982, p. 82). It is entirely possible, through intergenerational programming, that the nursing home may become the center of community involvement. For the children it becomes a living learning center, and for the elderly it becomes the new neighborhood. Gelfand also attests to the importance of neighborhood, at least for ethnic elderly, saying, "For ethnic older persons the neighborhood represents the site where much of their social interaction takes place and where the homes of a large proportion of their children, relatives, and friends are.   Dense ethnic communities provide elderly individuals with compatriots who share values, norms, and a common language" (1982, p. 51).

It is indeed a shame that, generally speaking, children in America are not afforded the opportunity to learn from the wisdom of neighborhood elderly but instead are age-segregated into public schools where the prime source of learning comes from textbook-guided curricula.

One alternative to age-segregated learning is the integration of school lessons into the activity programming of the nursing home and corresponding planning by the educational institution. Although educators and activities directors may be hesitant to embark on such an endeavor, the long-range gains far outweigh the extra time such planning might involve. In fact, both sides will find that preexisting activities easily complement each other, with elderly residents adding support to educational lessons and children offering an invaluable integration of laughter, smiles, ideas, questions, and overall warmth. Furthermore, the differentiation between age groups may not be so great as one might suspect. Children and elderly share a variety of concerns. "One common bond between the young child and the older person is the similar conditions they face. Both are socially disenfranchised, dependent upon 'significant others' for their needs, economically powerless, and subject to stereotypic representations" (M. Sorgman, M. Sorenson, and M. Johnston 1979, p. 135).

Pliny the Younger's *Letters* from the world of ancient Rome attest to the importance of intergenerational relationships. Though the manuscript supported understanding between the ages, there remained an outlook towards the aging process not unlike the one held by young people today. "On the one hand, Pliny philosophically looked forward to old age as that time of life when one is rewarded for past years of service. On the other hand, the *Letters* also hint that Pliny had not convinced himself that aging was a completely positive process" (R. Kebric 1983, p. 539). Pliny did, however, give readers the idea that there was a wealth of information to be learned from the elders. Sometimes the information passed on was purely academic in nature; at other times the data consisted of invaluable lessons regarding life skills. Thus, the intergenerational process is twofold, not only for passing on historical data, but also for day-to-day coping and survival skills. Coping with turn-of-the-century phases, new inventions, scientific discoveries, and economic changes are experiences elderly people are familiar with. Perhaps these experiences are the most important for children to learn about.

Mary Tyler John (1976, pp. 524-25) lists six important reasons for intergenerational education:

> 1. It seems important for children to learn that warm, sensitive relationships can span generations.
> 2. Children need to see age as a part of the total life cycle.
> 3. Learning about aging can help students face this phenomena more realistically.
> 4. It seems important, also, for children to learn about the contributions the older age group makes to our society. Knowing creative older individuals can give

young people a sense of hope and determination that is of great value to them.

5. Studying about the elderly can give the student a more positive picture of the total life span that will hopefully be available to him or her.

6. The elderly frequently demonstrate values and ideals that have survived the tests of time. Their sense of loyalty and commitment is inspirational to students on occasion.

Furthermore, the elderly may have more time to talk and listen to the problems or ideas of youth. In today's world of the working mother and father, it is often difficult for youths to find a good listening ear. The elderly may serve this purpose while at the same time enjoying the company of a newfound friend. Acquiring a sense of worth by contributing to the happiness and understanding of youth is vitally important to those who feel useless and forgotten.

The elderly generation becomes a "safe" sounding board for the adolescent as the fear of punishment is somewhat relieved. Students may go to a teacher, a counselor, or an administrator with problems, but all are indirectly connected with either an authoritative image or parents. The elderly, on the other hand, at the remove of a couple of generations, offer a nonthreatening opportunity for sharing problems or expressing ideas.

Older confidants may also offer years of life experience coping with problems, dealing with people, and surviving crises. Oncoming decades offer enormous personal, community, and world problems for the adolescent to solve. "It is known that divorce and drug abuse have traumatized recent generations of young people. In addition, the current generation of adolescents is anxious and insecure because of the escalation of nuclear technology and teen suicide. Children need role models who have conquered trauma and have gone on to embrace life with optimism" (J. Berkson and S. Griggs 1986, p. 140). The elderly, through their long survival, offer testimony that life goes on. Furthermore, the problems with which youth are confronted today may not be that different from those dealt with in earlier years by the elderly. Perhaps the current generation's problems seem more complicated or sophisticated, but the need to choose between right and wrong remains the same. Such basic emotions as love, fear, insecurity, sensitivity to peer pressure, and sadness exist no matter what the age or the scope of development in a culture. Our youngsters are confronted with some of the same primary concerns as were their grandparents. The danger lies, then, in not providing opportunities for youth to confront these problems and adequately develop problem-solving skills. "In our culture we tend to try to insulate the student from any and all of the real problems of life, and this constitutes a difficulty. It appears that if we desire to have students learn to be free and responsible individuals, then we must be willing for them to confront life, to face problems" (C. Rogers 1962, p. 10). By seeking advice and studying coping techniques used by the elderly, students can gain valuable knowledge to help them to realize successful solutions to their own problems.

The elderly also offer an invaluable resource for academic learning. Nancy Lubarsky combined a high school reading class with the elderly in an oral history project to study Halley's comet. "In this way they could compare life today to what it was like 75 years ago and, in doing so, learn about what changes have occurred. In addition, they would be able to use language in a variety of functions: to express their feelings and opinions about older people, to develop and clarify questions, to seek out information from guest speakers and reminiscences from the older people, to discuss what information should be included in the final project, and to write, edit, and revise the final publication" (N. Lubarsky 1987, p. 521).

It is not too far-fetched to speculate that someday the youth of America will be the immigrants of another planet. Shirley Polykoff in an interview in *More than Mere Survival* describes the belongings her immigrant parents brought to America. "They came here with a dowry: a straw satchel containing a feather bed, two pillows, one heavy Russian silver spoon and some dried fish" (J. Seskin 1980, p. 104). It is entirely possible that the youth of today may grow to be old immigrants travelling to another planet or space station where they too will carry with them only the bare necessities and a trinket as a remembrance of the homeland. What better preparation than the memory of their own great-great-grandparents or someone they have met who has made this same frightening but hopeful and exciting journey?

The therapeutic value of intergenerational programming for the elderly has been stated and restated in numerous research studies and in professional and personal testimonials. Maria McGovern of Luther Woods Convalescent Center gave her reaction to intergenerational programming: "The residents smile more often. Less complaints are heard about health problems. This type of ongoing affection turns the mind away from personal problems" (1980, p. 1).

The integration of youth and elderly, then, has implications that offer long-term impacts rather than short-lived results. Imagine the experience of talking with someone about Halley's comet and understanding their personal historical experience of it in the context of information about the period from various educational texts. This approach to learning from persons who have lived through it would come close to Hirsch's cultural learning. We have yet to include in our textbooks valuable interviews with persons who have lived through historical moments. Where are textbook questions asking how old were you when this happened? How did you feel? How did you react? How did it change your life? Before the fragmentation of the family, youngsters could ask their grandparents; now it is up to society to find avenues to link this oral living history to the overall educational experience of our youngsters. Contact with the elderly makes sense out of history, reason out of relationships, and rhyme out of life.

A second component that deserves investigation is the impact of the arts on youth and the elderly. We are speaking of arts as areas of activity that help individuals to create, express, and communicate ideas, including drama, music, movement and dance, visual arts, writing, and reading interpretation.

THE NEED FOR ARTS EXPERIENCES

The arts have been used for expression and communication throughout the centuries. One can trace the early forms of the expressive arts through ritualism and even in therapy. As the Feders point out, "Pythagoras, the mathematician-physician, used dance and music with mental patients. He introduced a theory of psychobiosis, in which music (which he called 'musical medicine') played a central role in promoting order, proportion, and measure" (1981, p. 4).

Ancient civilizations used art as a means to bring about a change, to record an episode, or to communicate a need. This becomes very clear in watching the National Folkloric Ballet of Mexico, where one particular choreographed piece represents the ancient culture's experience in hunting deer. The movements of the dancer representing the deer are at first careful and calculated, but as the tension builds, the motions become frenetic with fear and excitement as the pursuer closes the distance between hunter and hunted.

We study the artifacts and artwork of ancient cultures to find out what they did, how they did, and, we hope, why they did it. It is usually through the arts that we find records of history, of culture, and of traditions. On a recent trip to Chichen Itza in Mexico, I looked with awe at one of the ancient Mayan performance platforms and thought how careful we are to learn from ancient civilizations, yet how careless in gathering information from our current "ancients," the elderly.

It makes sense, then, to study the art of the elderly and to offer them avenues of expression and communication that may not have been available to them. It makes sense also to involve youth, who will make the most use of the information gained in developing an intelligent and artistic civilization, sensitive to the values of nature and mankind. Through this ancient expressive tool of the arts, the elder generation may communicate with the younger generation to pass on knowledge, explore new avenues, and discover dormant talents.

Another "general population" art-process exists, unmeasured but necessary for the well-being of a culture. Artists are able to express for us what we think we may not have the time or talent to express. Comedy clubs take on a new significance during an age of concerns over nuclear war, unsolved diseases, and yet-to-be-understood intelligence. The importance of super-hero films is magnified when the culture feels a need to solve pressing problems but lacks the vital threads to unravel the mysteries and untangle the disputes. By attending films, we may live vicariously through the successful endeavors of Superman and Batman. These fantasy adventures let us enter into "safe" combat with the evil forces and prevail. There is a sense of community art in the audience, which is later carried home, if not by the adults, then certainly by the children.

The opportunity for art experiences is more prevalent in today's education than it was for the elderly. There still remain needs to express, to explore, to invent, and certainly to dream. "Remember also that the creating of images has been a basic mode of communication for man since primeval times. And because such symbolic visual power is universal and is still alive today, we are able to encourage the release of spontaneous expression in new ways in order to develop fresh forms of human adjustment" (M. Naumburg 1964, p. 221). Bob Fleshman and Jerry L. Fryrear continue this theme in stating, "The arts therapies have mainly been used to help non-artists, average people who have not developed most of the artistic potentials within them. Arts therapists help them to fulfill this potential through the use of the materials and methods of the arts and by stimulating greater creativity within them" (1981, p. 6). Michael Kirby gives a succinct definition of Moreno's psychodrama in stating that "the concern is not with 'good theatre' as a result or product but with the psychological benefits to the performer of acting in certain ways" (1976, p. 3).

The arts, then, whether as therapy or as, entertainment, help individuals to express, imagine, and communicate in a unique manner. One is never too young or too old to learn to communicate through the arts. "Even the finest intellect is part of a being who has also five major senses and imagination; the intellect will not be harmed by fully developing the senses and the imagination, and the uses to which that intellect are eventually put may well depend, in human terms, on precisely imagination and an acute sensitivity" (Brian Way 1967, p. 64). In discussing the importance of visual arts experiences, Lorraine Lauzon says, "Age is no criteria in the world of art. Whether it be the age of the masterpiece or the artist himself, when the young and old get together artistically, the results can be dynamic" (1981, p. 41). Liz Lerman's Dance Exchange Program and Dancers of the Third Age (P. McCutcheon and C. Wolf 1985, p. 136) modern dance troupe for senior citizens "demonstrates the belief that dance as an art form can bring health, vitality, self-understanding, and a sense of belonging to older people, and that this contact with the elderly contributes to the artistic development of the younger dancer" (1981, p. 19-20).

It has been reported that the importance of arts in public education has been undermined for years, yet as one travels across the United States, discrepencies in the support of arts studies becomes apparent.   Some geographical areas may fully support arts programs; others because of funding difficulties or disagreement as to the necessity of such learning, may offer few or no art experiences. Greg Snider attributes some of the decline of interest in the arts to governments and institutions of higher learning.   "The rationalization of education insists, as part of its platform, that all available programs form part of a larger interlocking whole, not only with the hierarchy of primary, secondary and post-secondary education within a province, but finally within a national scheme that standardizes and conforms education to a goal-oriented model of corporate and industrial accommodation in the name of efficiency" (1985, pp. 3-4). Although it is difficult in the late 1980s and early 1990s to argue with the supply-and-demand theory of education and the consequent employment of our students, it is necessary to study the effects of the lack of arts training or appreciation in their studies. The arts offer a look at the culture, a study of the expression of the times, and a moment of self-reflection if the viewer has the background training to see all that is being said, sung, danced, or painted.   If, however, the individual is not attuned to interpretation or examination or, for that matter, the use of the imagination, the work is lost and the viewer may have missed an important interpretation, which affects his life, his business, and his world. Therefore, art programs and the subsequent training of artists are important to the well-being and development of individuals. "The role of any art program is to clarify for the artists within what they are doing and why, so that their intentionality is not misconstrued. The arts have a fundamental stake in this encouragement, and their continued survival is not a question of self-interest, but of the importance of their ability to bring artists to full consciousness of the meaning and consequence of their acts and their ideas. For culture itself, this means a critical presence that can freely examine the suppositions and premises on which that culture is based" (Snider 1985, p. 5).

Somewhere among art therapy, art appreciation, and formal art training lies applied art, that which may combine therapy, training, and appreciation for a holistic experience. Here, there may or may not be a final performance, painting, or story, because the experience is valued for the process rather than the product. Through the process, one experiences with all the senses and appreciates the opportunity to be a part of a new dimension. The applied arts are exploratory, imaginative, and investigative and offer to the participant the opportunity to reflect and respond without the fear of failure or criticism.   Rather than being limited by an audition, drawing, or portfolio submission, the applied arts are available to all who wish to participate, regardless of age, training, or proven talent.

APPLIED ARTS AND INTERGENERATIONAL PROGRAMMING

The combined efforts of applied art and intergenerational programming may offer both individual and collective development toward a better understanding of humanity and its surroundings. The elderly may gain a better understanding of youth, thereby enabling them to communicate with and to assist a generation in moving forward. The youth benefit from the life skills and academic knowledge of the elderly and thereby become better prepared to deal with living. "One way in which the child can explore the past, appreciate the present, and forecast his or her future is through exploring the concept of ageism" (M. Sorgman, M. Sorenson, and M. Johnston 1979, p. 138).

Intergenerational arts programming, then, offers an opportunity for individual development and expression combined with collective learning through working together. It is humanistic learning by doing, and what better way is there to bring the generations together, thus developing an intergenerational culture?

HELPFUL TEXTS

Balkema, John B. 1986. *The Creative Spirit: An Annotated Bibliography on the Arts, Humanities and Aging.* Washington, D.C.: National Council on the Aging.

Lewis-Kane, M., P. McCutcheon, and R. MacDicken. 1986. *Arts Mentor Program: A Manual for Sponsors.* Washington, D.C.: National Council on the Aging.

McCutcheon, P. 1986. *An Arts and Aging Media Sourcebook: Films, Videos, Slide/Tape Shows.* Washington, D.C.: National Council on the Aging.

McCutcheon, P. 1986. *A Manual for Artists: How to Find Work in the Field of Aging.* Washington, D.C.: National Council on the Aging.

McCutcheon, P., and C. Wolf. 1985. *The Resource Guide to People, Places, and Programs in Arts and Aging.* Washington, D.C.: National Council on the Aging.

Ross, L., and G. Beall. *Intergenerational Programming: Opportunities for National Organizations.* Washington,D.C.: National Council on the Aging.

Ventura-Merkel, C. 1988. *Planning a Family Friends Project: A Working Guide.* Volume 12. Washington, D.C.: National Council on the Aging.

REFERENCES

Bausell, R., A. Rooney, and C. Inlander. 1988. *How to Evaluate and Select a Nursing Home*. New York: Addison-Wesley Publishing Company.

Berkson, J., and S. Griggs. 1986. "An Intergenerational Program at a Middle School." *The School Counselor* 34:140-43.

Cetron, M., B. Soriano, and M. Gale. 1985. *Schools of the Future: How American Business Can Cooperate to Save Our Schools*. New York: McGraw-Hill Book Company.

Feder, E., and B. Feder. 1981. *The Expressive Arts Therapies: Art, Music, and Dance As Psychotherapy*. New York: Prentice-Hall, Inc.

Fleshman, B., and J. L. Fryrear. 1981. *The Arts in Therapy*. Chicago: Nelson Hall.

Gelfand, Donald E. 1982. *Aging: The Ethnic Factor*. Boston: Little, Brown and Company.

Halpern, James. 1987. *Helping Your Aging Parents*. New York: Fawcett Press.

Hickey, T., L. Hickey, and R. Kalish. 1968. "Children's Perceptions of the Elderly." *The Journal of Genetic Psychology* 112:227-235.

Hirsch, E. D., Jr. 1987. *Cultural Literacy: What Every American Needs To Know*. Boston: Houghton Mifflin Company.

John, M. 1977. "Teaching Children about Older Family Members." *Social Education* 41:524-27.

Kebric, R. 1983. "Aging in Pliny's *Letters*: A View from the Second Century A.D." *The Gerontologist* 23:538-45.

Kirby, Michael. 1976. "Introduction." *The Drama Review* 20:3.

Lauzon, L. 1981. "Art Project Spans the Generations." *Design for Arts in Education* 83:41-3.

Lerman, L. and C. Reeverts. 1981. "The Dance Exchange." *Design for Arts in Education* 83:11-20.

Lubarsky, N. 1987. "A Glance at the Past, a Glimpse of the Future." *Journal of Reading* 30:520-29.

McCutcheon, P., and C. Wolf. 1985. *The Resource Guide to People, Places, and Programs in Arts and Aging*. Washington, D.C.: National Council on the Aging.

McGovern, M. 1983. "The Young Keep the Fun in Growing Old." " Activity Director's Guide." 10 Mimeo.

Naumburg, M. 1977. "Spontaneous Art in Education and Psychotherapy." In *Art Therapy in Theory and Practice*, 2nd ed., edited by E. Ulman and P. Dachinger, 221-22. New York: Shocken Books.

Powell, J., and G. Arquitt. 1978. "Getting the Generations Back Together: A Rationale for Development of Community Based Intergenerational Interaction Programs." *The Family Coordinator* 27:421-26.

Rogers, C. 1962. "Learning to Be Free," Paper given to a session on "Conformity and Diversity" in the conference on "Man and Civilization," University of California, School of Medicine, San Francisco, 28 January 1962.

Seskin, J. 1980. *More than Mere Survival*: *Conversations with Women over 65*. New York: Newsweek Books.

Snider, G. 1985. "The Future of Arts Education." excerpted from a paper presented at a panel discussion on "Art and the Universities," Contemporary Art Gallery, Vancouver, B. C., 28 November 1984.

Sorgman, M., M. Sorenson, and M. Johnston. 1979. "What Sounds Do I Make When I'm Old?" *Social Education* 43:135-39.

Way, Brian. 1967. *Development through Drama*. New York: Humanities Press.

2

Successful Intergenerational Programming

Since 1980, a number of intergenerational programs and organizations have evolved at local, regional, and national levels. Generations United, a national coalition on intergenerational issues and programs, states the following as its purpose:

> . To unite at national, state and local levels on key public policy issues that address human needs across all generations.

> . To increase awareness of the public and the Coalition members' constituents of the common issues faced by Americans of every generation.

> . To produce and disseminate programmatic information and materials for the member organizations, their constituents and the public that demonstrate the value of intergenerational cooperation and stimulate such cooperation. (Generations United 1990)

Another significant development has been that of the Intergenerational Program at the National Council on the Aging (NCOA) and the subsequent publication of *Growing Together: An Intergenerational Sourcebook* (K. Struntz 1985) published by the American Association of Retired Persons (AARP). The NCOA has become a national resource for listings of programs, bibliographies, ideas, and support.

It is helpful to study the descriptions of various programs evolved over the last decade, some of which still thrive, some of which lasted for a specified length of time, and others that continue to grow, change, and evolve. Not all of the programs described here are based in nursing homes, yet all are adaptable in some way to the long-term health care facility. Just as the projects suggest diverse program designs, one must keep in mind that even nursing home populations are diverse in their makeup, administration, and overall design. Practitioners should study each program and consider the population with whom they are serving and working.

Included in this overview are educational programs based in social studies, home economics, social skills, and history that lend themselves to the arts and language arts. During the ten-year interval, many school districts have developed curriculum guides helpful in organizing and designing appropriate units of study for various states and educational regions. The National Council on the Aging offers an excellent resource guide, *Community Planning for Intergenerational Programming*, Volume 8 (C. Ventura-Merkel and L. Lidoff 1983), which leads practioners and interested participants through the steps in the development and implementation of intergenerational programming.

The listings and descriptions are by no means definitive. The programs discussed are ones the author felt most useful in local schools and nursing homes. All of the programs seem to share in what Catherine Ventura-Merkel and Lorraine Lidoff describe as "common themes of success" :

. A systematic process of development

. Leadership strongly committed to seeing
the program take root and succeed

. Core staff with a strong commitment

. Involvement of potential partners

. Adequate resources...(1983, p. ii)

The programs share another element for success, that of collaborative investigation. Discoveries are made daily concerning human relationships and the complexity of successful communication between ages and groups. Thus, programs begun in the 1970s may take on a new flavor as we communicate in the 1990s and implement them with a different set of children, those who are now involved in an era of fast-paced information reception and retrieval.

One final consideration brings great hope as we begin our progression through the 1990s. This final hope is Carolyn Corbin's suggestion that "the trend in the New Age Economy will be to help the individual relate to other people better. With people having much of the manual labor done for them, and even many of their mental efforts replaced by computers, for the first time in American history, in fact in world history, we will be resolved to relate. This will be one of the most profound effects of the New Age Economy" (1989, p. 30). If Corbin's predictions are correct, what better time than now to look at past, present, and future programs which bring together our most powerful resource, humanity?

EXAMPLES OF SUCCESSFUL PROGRAMMING

As early as 1978, Judith Powell and George Arquitt reported that in one intergenerational project in which students learned about history, "Older adults were more successful than classroom teachers in teaching preschool children how ways of living change, and how people change over time" (p. 423).

Margo Sorgman;, Marilou Sorenson, and Marilyn Johnston developed an excellent lesson in social studies for grades four through six. "These activities are based on such key social studies concepts as change, culture, values, individualism, and futurism; and they reflect an interdisciplinary approach to social studies" (1979, p. 135). Such exercises as "Culture Creatures," in which students compare and contrast the cultures and traditions of older people, and "Corner Conversations," in which students become social scientists by collecting and analyzing data about the life-styles of older people, provide opportunities for interaction with the elderly in the community or in the nursing home.

James Hauwiller and Russell Jennings (1981) actually took gerontology into the classrooms of second, third, and fourth graders in Montana. Their teachers were given pre-workshop inservice training in an effort to dispel stereotypical views they might hold about the aging. They were asked to review teaching texts for references to the elderly and were invited to develop lessons that would counteract negative views and support positive ones. They were also provided with a manual (J. Hauwiller, R. Jennings, and G. Refsland 1978) to assist the teaching of gerontological topics along with conventional school subjects. Children involved in creative writing exercises were motivated by such topics as "My Favorite Aged Person" and "Everyone Thought She Was Crabby." They were also provided with learning center experiences such as creating of a collage illustrating the activities of older people.

Hauwiller and Jennings reported in their findings not only that the students' views of aging had improved but also that because of this educational experience in gerontology the children learned that "the aged are as varied in interests, abilities, health, mobility, and other traits as are other groups in society. This alternate view holds potential to counteract the more simplistic idea of the aged that children might get from knowledge only of grandparents or what is learned on the once a year trip to the retirement home" (p.189).

In an intergenerational art project conducted by Lorraine Lauzon at the Berkshire Museum in Pittsfield, Massachusetts, children illustrated the reminiscences of the elderly. In describing the project Lauzon explains:

> After the collected memories were typed on separated sheets of paper, I asked the children, whose ages range from 6 to 12, to illustrate the thoughts and ideas.   The illustrations were done with crayons, watercolor, or pen and ink. The results were delightful. The stories were purposely kept short and in simple language, so the children could easily interpret them. Some stories were in the form of poetry. (1981, p. 41)

The collected memories of the elderly were as rich in images as were the imaginations of the children. Such topics as new Easter clothes, ethnic traditions, and specific religious themes were suggested by the Supportive Services coordinator, Merlyn Girard.

> A gentleman originally from New Orleans described an exciting Easter-egg cracking game he remembered playing with his brother. There were memories of sumptuous holiday feasts, and even a treasured family recipe for Polish cookies. (I ran off copies of this for the children, so they could have their mothers bake them.) (p.41)

Information exchange may flow in the opposite direction as well. Children are and will become excellent resources for sharing information with those removed from the mainstream of education. "For a child who is ten years old today, there will be four times as much knowledge available to that child when he goes to college as is available to him now" (C. Corbin 1989, p. 26).

In her article "Teaching Children about Older Family Members", Martha Tyler John describes activities involving cross-generational exchange. In this article the author recognizes the value in lifelong learning. "Elderly people need to continue to learn, and there are some skills and information that students in elementary school possess that could be shared with an older individual who learned under a different system or setting. To promote a feeling of mutual give-and-take to provide stimulation for the older person, the author recommends that students tutor the older person on occasion" (1977, p. 527). Some interesting tutorial programs described in her article involve the metric system, the use of media, and a "Good Old Days" program.

Project Teen-Ager in South Carolina (Morris, Judson 1984) enabled adolescents and the elderly to exchange skills and knowledge while improving the quality of life and self-esteem of both groups. Sixty students from Manning High School worked with residents at South Carolina Community Long Term Care, a state agency for elderly persons who need assistance to remain at home. Teams of four students to one elderly person worked on such activities as "gardening, housekeeping, cooking, helping with school homework, transporting, talking, and listening."

NUTRITION AND INTERGENERATIONAL LEARNING

Another project that successfully united the talents of seniors and adolescents was that of Channel One in Rochester, Minnesota (Allen 1986). Originally intended as an effort to prevent drug abuse among adolescents in the area, the program reached far beyond its major goal by bringing together the generations to raise funds for, manage, and share in the experience of a food co-op for senior citizens. Adolescents also served as members of the board of directors, which gave them a sense of self-worth and importance. An adolescent and a senior gave testimonials at the Senate Select Committee on Aging. One 18-year-old student's reaction to her involvement with the food co-op was as follows:

> I just never had the chance before to really meet older people. When you're my age, you don't get the opportunity to sit down and talk with people who have lived a lot longer than you....I look at myself very differently now. This experience has added so much more to me, to my understanding. It has opened my eyes and changed my life. (p. 34)

The reaction of a 66-year-old volunteer provided further insight into this project:

> It helps seniors but it also brings people together-the old and the young. I think that's important because youngsters don't have older people to be with usually and this kind of gives them grandparents who

care....Older people need affection. And most young
people can be very affectionate and caring....It is also
very rewarding to watch the young people who help the
elderly and see how much they get out of it and how
good it makes them feel to serve someone else. (p.34)

Project MAIN (Mobile Assistants in Nutrition) exemplifies a
collaborative effort shared by a senior service agency, a university, and a high
school to "research, plan and operate a grocery delivery and escort service for
the elderly and disabled residents living in a targeted neighborhood" (G. Blake
1986, p. 32). The students were paid through grants, and private foundations
provided the necessary financial assistance for this project in Oregon, which
the Youth Employment Planning Team at Portland State University designed.
The project also included interrelated studies for the students in gerontology,
interpersonal communications, disability awareness, the economics of food
shopping, and nutrition. Students were able to obtain both academic and
work-experience credit for their active participation in Project MAIN. Gerald
F. Blake desribes the educational component in the following manner:

The students heard lectures, completed individual
reading assignments, participated in small group
discussions, visited senior service agencies, and received
training in the use of wheelchairs and other mobility
devices. (p.33)

The impact of the project was immense, with the youth serving 238
elderly and disabled persons over a twelve-month period, while logging 1,560
shopping and escort trips to grocery stores. The project helped students to
"gain valuable work experience, explore a variety of human service careers, and
learn a considerable amount about nutrition, disabilities, and aging. In
addition, the relationships that were established between the youths and the
elderly proved to be much stronger and more enduring than was anticipated.
Several students continued to visit and shop for their elderly clients even after
the project ended" (p.33).

It is important to note that this particular project was a collaborative
effort, involving three major institutions in the community: agencies serving the
aging, public schools, and universities. All too often these institutions work
separately in the community without using their abundant resources to achieve
goals. All communities should be encouraged to work on projects that
combine the talents and resources of various institutions. Working
relationships between universities and public schools are of vital importance, as
many students are affected by the conduct of research universities but are not
actively involved in the results. Blake concludes that "the Mobile Assistants in

Nutrition project demonstrates that universities, high schools and social service agencies can collaborate to produce solutions to community problems that are academically relevant, enhance the transition from school to work and improve the quality of communities" (p. 34).

This program might be revised in such a way that high school students would shop for nursing home residents. Such programs may also develop into performance art projects enabling students to learn about effective shopping and servicing.

A suggestion for integrating nutrition education with the arts is given through the dramatization of the play *Meals on Wheels* (J. Orlock, nd R. Cornish 1976). Barbara W. Davis supports the use of this particular play for its educational and humanistic value to participants and audience members. In her article "Drama: A Tool for Nutrition Education with Older Adults," she discusses a project that used this play as a catalyst for nutrition education and discussion. She described the positive impact in the following manner: "Psychological conditions can have a powerful influence on the nutritional well-being of individuals, but effectively explaining or describing this influence is often difficult. Drama holds promise as a medium through which we can convey the impact of psychological conditions on nutrition" (1983, p. 5).

It may be possible for teenagers from a high school to become involved in a production of this short play as actors, directors, or set designers. Again, the education would be twofold, as both elderly people and youth would learn through the process of production and discussion. A play of this type would also easily support studies in a home economics class.

Penny A. Ralston et al. (1986) have prepared a curriculum guide for the integration of aging education into the secondary home economics class. The working guide is divided into four major units of study, including (1) perceptions of older people and the aging process, (2) biological/physiological aspects of aging, (3) demographic trends of aging, and (4) intergenerational communication. Writing logs and creative writing activities related to feelings and observations about aging included in this guide help to promote across-the-curriculum writing. A further step might be to have the elderly keep either written or tape-recorded logs of their feelings about the youths. The guide is also very helpful in listing and describing several curriculum sources in home economics and gerontology that are desiged for classroom use at the elementary and high school levels.

A combination of this guide and a production of *Meals on Wheels* (J. Orlock and R. Cornish 1976) would certainly provide both the high school class and the community agency with a well-rounded experience in nutrition, communication, socialization, and artistic expression.

Various educational districts have also become excellent resources for the integration of intergenerational programming.

CALIFORNIA'S INTERGENERATIONAL PROGRAMMING

The California State Department of Education published "Young and Old Together: A Resource Directory of Intergenerational Programs in 1985. The directory listings provide such information as descriptions of programs, funding sources, and addresses of intergenerational projects. Of particular interest to primary and secondary teachers is Project Joy, which "introduces students in private and public schools to older people in the community who live in senior centers and nursing homes to promote mutual respect, understanding, and friendship between the generations. The project involves an in-depth aging awareness curriculum, regular visits to senior centers and nursing homes, an intergenerational summer camp, older guests sharing stories about their lives in the classroom, and in-service education for teachers and parents" (p.4).

Programs designed for high school students included the Intergenerational Program at Adelante High School, where throughout the school year students distributed holiday cards that they designed to convalescing seniors. The Audubon Junior High School and Crenshaw/Manual Arts High Schools were involved in lessons on aging and power-writing techniques. "Students apply their writing skills to the lessons taught for articles for the 'Dialogue' newsletter, which is published periodically" (p.9).

Students at A.G. Currie Intermediate School have participated in the Courtesy Card Program, volunteering their services at a home for the elderly, Tustin Manor. This program is unique in that "a 'courtesy card' is issued to a student when he or she performs an act of service. After 15 cards are awarded to a student, he or she is presented with a large framed certificate during a special assembly, thus providing recognition and reinforcement of positive student behavior" (p.8). At Pueblo Vista Elementary School "fourth, fifth, and sixth graders from the Learning Lab for Gifted Students are divided in S.A.G.E. Committees (Students Aware of Growing Elderly) whose goal is to complete a report on various aspects of aging. The goal is not to accumulate facts but to heighten students' awareness of the problems, joys, and inevitability of aging" (pp.1-2).

Probably one of the most interesting names was that of SWING (Seniors with Interests in New Generations) who work in conjunction with Workman Elementary School in La Puente, California. This program is "designed to recognize the importance of and provide a reciprocal community-wide opportunity for interaction between seniors and elementary schoolchildren. Particular emphasis is placed on involving schools with limited-English-proficient children" (p. 15).

The resource directory lists thirty-five intergenerational programs that took place or are currently taking place in the California Public Schools. One of the projects, the Courtesy Card Program at A.G. Currie Intermediate School, has been in existence since 1974. The success of intergenerational programming in California has also generated a *Handbook for Instruction on Aging*, with curriculum guides for kindergarten through the twelfth grade (1978). The handbook includes five content areas of instruction on aging, including (1) Chronological Aging, (2) Physiological/Biological Aging, (3) Sociocultural Aspects of Aging, (4) Psychological Aging, and (5) The Commmunity and the Older Individual. Furthermore, each content area includes suggested objectives for elementary (kindergarten through grade six) or secondary (grades seven through twelve) levels. The Glossary of Terms at the back of the handbook is especially helpful to teachers and may provide classes with vocabulary and spelling words. An intergenerational spelling bee using these words and terms might prove interesting, as the words stir response and might motivate discussion concerning denotation and connotation.

SUCCESSFUL PROGRAMMING AROUND THE COUNTRY

Involving seniors with learning-disabled junior and senior high school students in Redding, Connecticut, proved successful for both age groups. Seniors developed games to help improve the academic skills of the students rather than taking on a traditional didactic relationship. Positive outcomes included achievement in academic skills and improvement in outlook toward school, and parents reported favorable behavioral and attitudinal changes (R. Drummond et al. 1975).

Eighth graders from the Jones-Village Partnership Program in Columbus, Ohio, spent their English and history classes at a nearby retirement center, First Community Village, and enriched their learning by talking with the elderly, taping oral histories, and keeping daily journals (J. Firman and A. Stowell 1980). Similar projects have appeared nationwide in an effort to provide students with "living-learning" rather than to limit their knowledge to textbook studies. James Firman and Anita Stowell support integenerational programming in high schools, stating that "educators have a responsibility to help students understand the process and phenomenon of aging in our society, and to provide them with opportunities to learn with and from older people. American high schools are a fertile environment for experimenting and pioneering intergenerational programs" (pp.19,42).

One program that focused on performance art was conducted at Mt. View Elementary School, where students were exposed to various cross sections of the elderly population of the community through dance. Students visited a nursing home and a retirement hotel and participated in dance with the elderly in their own classroom. The culminating activity was a celebration in which "dance, art, poetry, and journal entries that had taken place throughout the week were performed, displayed or presented to each other and to the guest of honor Aunt Sally Williams -- who was 100 years old" (J. Metal-Corbin, D. Corbin, and G. Barker 1986, pp. 7-8). A videotape of this process is available through the University of Nebraska at Omaha (Bottum et al. 1985).

An early childhood intervention program (M. Dellmann-Jenkins, D. Lambert, and D. Fruit 1986) proved successful at Kent State University, where 3 and 4-year-olds involved in a university-based day care center were given the opportunity to interact with older volunteer teaching assistants, senior citizens participating in a local day care center for adults, and curriculum materials and activities that promoted positive intergenerational experiences. Many of the arts activities involving seniors and the children included music, art, and dramatic play. Dramatic play, it should be mentioned at this point, is an important developmental stage in a child's growth and a beginning for the child's continued growth towards creative dramatics, role-playing, formal drama, and dramatic problem-solving.

The state of Pennsylvania, long recognized as a leader in the field of intergenerational programming, developed a program that assists different agencies to correlate projects be beneficial both to young children and to seniors (C. Lyons 1986). The program was "conceived and implemented in Pennsylvania by Generations Together, a program of the University of Pittsburgh Center for Social and Urban Research entitled 'Developing Intergenerational Programs Jointly with the Aging and Child Care Networks in Pennsylvania' " (p.22). It is significant that by the end of the project one objective, to develop approximately fifty intergenerational programs throughout the state involving both the elderly and young children, had been expanded to aim for sixty-four programs. One example of programming involved children and seniors in music, art, and movement activities. The testimonial of one teacher sums up the positive outcome of this project: "It is a shot in the arm for caring teachers to watch the faces of young and old light up as they grow to care about each other" (p. 23).

A program that received the "Best Intergenerational Showcase Award" from the American Association on Aging, for 1985-86 was the Grandparent, Read to Me Project at the Lakewood Preschool for learning-disabled children 3 to 5 years old, in Lakewood, Ohio. An important point made by this program and by the author who was Coordinator of Special Programs for the Lakewood City Schools (Jones, 1986) was that preschoolers may become confused by the difference between paternal or maternal grandparents and grandparent tutors, thereby necessitating some pre-project tutoring. One pre-project arts activity, the creation of a family collage, included the children's own grandparents. The results of this program stressed the improved interest in books on the part of the children, as reported not only by the teacher but by the parents as well. An added dimension best depicted by the author, describing the culminating activity of the project, was an intergenerational field trip to a children's farm and subsequent picnic:

> The farm was selected because it coincided with the content of several of the stories the children had enjoyed. Also, many of the senior volunteers had lived in the country and felt this would be a positive experience for the urban students. At the end of the day the volunteers presented each student with a copy of a selected book as a remembrance. The preschoolers gave each volunteer a plastic mug they had colored as a thank-you. (p.37)

The benefits of the elderly as child care helpers or providers should also be examined, for child care offers opportunities that reach beyond the child and help the working parent or parents who are in need of high-quality childcare but may lack the funds to seek out private day care or do not qualify for government-subsidized day care. The Lucy Corr Nursing Home in Chesterfield, Virginia, is a long-term care facility that offers child care programming. According to Judy Beach, Activities Director, the value of such a program to both seniors and the children is immeasurable (P. Clark 1989). Seniors look forward to the visitation period, and children enter with open arms, laughter, warm smiles, and a generally optimistic outlook on life. Marilyn J. Miller further supports this concept in examining the amount of time children spend in the child care setting. "The presence of elderly adults can have a significant effect on the development of positive attitudes toward such persons and toward the aging process" (1986, pp. 158-59). The process of touching is also supported by Miller as an aspect that may be lost to the elderly because of the death of a spouse or isolation from children and grandchildren. It is yet another contribution children can make in this setting.

Through the University of Pittsburgh, high school students from economically distressed families in the Steel Valley are afforded the opportunity to work with frail institutionalized and homebound older persons in the community. A curriculum, "Perspectives on Aging," has been developed, and further expansion to include students in grades nine through eleven and the seventh and eighth grade middle school band and art classes was planned (J. Kenny 1988). This particular program is supported by VISTA and Student Community Service programs.

Camp Fire, Inc., offers guidance for intergenerational involvement through a program entitled "Friendship across the Ages." This program is important to study because it offers yet another avenue for participation. This past year one of my high school students approached me with the idea of earning a badge for her scout troop by working with me on a weekly basis at the nursing home. She became instrumental in the planning and implementation of the drama program and will continue her work during the 1990-91 school year, long after earning her award. One of the most touching and rewarding moments came during the summer, when she visited the nursing home dressed in full uniform, proudly displaying the badges she had earned over the years and giving the residents special thanks for her most recent badge, which they had helped her to acquire. The moment of applause was indeed a special moment of mutual respect and pride.

The brochure received from Camp Fire, Inc., as recently as August of 1990 offers guidance for students involved in this program, yet the information is helpful to anyone interested in working and sharing across the generations. The following steps are listed for the "Friendship across the Ages" participant:

1. Make a Time Commitment of
   Six Months.

2. Learn about Aging

3. Give Service.

4. Communicate.

5. Share a Meal.

6. Learn Life Stories.

7. Celebrate the Friendship.

8. Record the Experience.
   (p.2)

Of special interest to language arts teachers is the section concerning communication and ideas for letter writing, notecards, journal writing, and story writing. The brochure also lists books and films appropriate for grades one through nine.

Another brochure received this summer from the Danbury School in Claremont, California, concerned its incorporation of older volunteers to assist with orthopedically handicapped students. "The presence of volunteers decreases the pupil/adult ratio and allows teachers more time to interact with students on an individual basis" (Danbury School Intergenerational Program).

Recent communication with Kansas State University's Cooperative Extension Service revealed three resource guides for Grandletters, described as "a correspondence program for grandparents and their grandchildren" (C. Smith and G. Gutsch 1985). Language arts teachers and activities directors will find this series, which includes "Grandchild Letters," instructions for the students, "Grandparent Letters," instructions for the grandparent, and "Program Instructions," helpful in participating in such a program. Through the exchange of ten key letters, participants focus upon the following issues:

> Affection and friendship
> Family and heritage
> Generosity and love
> Responsibility and courage
> Respect for elders
> Honesty and commitment
> Helpfulness
> Competition and justice
> Conflict and violence
> Sadness and grief. (p.1)

All of these topics would of course lend themselves to investigation through dance, music, and drama as well as writing.

A second publication, "Generations Together," from Kansas State University, provides a guide for ten visits between the generations, using the ten previously listed issues as the focal point. Teachers will be interested in the Grandbook and Journal assignments. The publication is written for the elderly participant and provides a step-by-step review of the process, including goals and activities for each visit. The diverse activities range from making no-bake cookies and the sharing of a snack to visual arts activities. Although this publication is currently out of print, interested participants may obtain photocopies from the Cooperative Extension Service at Kansas State University.

Yet another way of bringing the generations together is through a program held yearly since 1986 in Tampa, Florida. Program Director Anne Justiss describes Intergenerational Day as "a festival which combines old and young in a day of play using the creative arts and other forms of unconventional therapy to jump the generational barrier and bridge the generational gap" (Justiss 1990).

The list of intergenerational programming is growing, giving strong testimony to the value of such endeavors. One can see from the descriptions of some of the programs, both the past and present, that they reach a very diverse population and may be housed and designed in any number of ways to fit the needs of the participants. In the face of such support, growth, and enthusiasm, it is difficult to argue against such project ideas; instead we should look toward a stong movement in education to get the generations back together and allow all to participate in lifelong learning and understanding.

HELPFUL ADDRESSES AND CONTACTS

American Association of Retired Persons
1909 K Street, N.W.
Washington, D.C. 20049

California State Department of Education
721 Capitol Mall
Sacramento, California 95814-4785

Camp Fire, Inc.
"Friendship across the Ages"
4601 Madison Avenue
Kansas City, Missouri 64112-1278

Danbury School for Orthopedically Handicapped
Danbury School Intergenerational Program
Arnold Bloom, Principal
1700 Danbury Road
Claremont, California 91711

Generations United
c/o Child Welfare League of America, Inc.
440 First Street, N.W., Suite 310
Washington, D.C. 20001-2085

Kansas State University
Cooperative Extension Service
"Grandletters"
"Generations Together"
Manhattan, Kansas 66506

National Council on the Aging, Inc.
600 Maryland Avenue, S.W.
West Wing 100
Washington, D.C. 20024

REFERENCES

Allen, M.   1986.   "Channel One: An Intergenerational Program at Work."
    Children Today 15 (3):32-34.
Blake, G. 1986. "Project MAIN: Classwork in the Community Benefits Senior
    Citizens." *Children Today* 15 (4):31-34.
Bottum, D. (producer/director), J. Metal-Corbin, G. Barker (project
    directors), and D. Corbin (narrator/writer). 1985. *Age Doesn't
    Matter: Weaving Dance and Aging into a Fifth Grade Curriculum.*
    Videotape.   Omaha: University Television,   University of
    Nebraska at Omaha.
Clark, P. 1989.   Interview with Judy Beach, Activities Director, Lucy Corr
    Nursing Home, Chesterfield, Virginia.
Corbin, C. 1989. *Strategies 2000: How to Prosper in the New Age.* Austin, Tex.:
    Eakin Press.
"Danbury School Intergenerational Program." Danbury School, 1700 Danbury
    Road, Claremont, California, 91711.
Davis, B. 1983. "Drama: A Tool for Nutrition Education with Older Adults."
    Journal of Nutrition Education 15:5
Dellman-Jenkins, M., D. Lambert, and D. Fruit.   1986.   "Old and Young
    Together: Effect of an Educational Program on Preschoolers'
    Attitudes Toward Older People." *Childhood Education* 63:206-
    212.
Drummond, R., et al. 1975. "Project STEP (Seniors Tutor for Educational
    Progress)." On-Site Validation Report, Easton-Redding Regional
    School District 9, Connecticut.
Firman, J., and A. Stowell.   1980.   "Intergenerational School Projects:
    Examples and Guidelines." *Media and Methods* 17:19,42.
"Friendship across the Ages." 1984. Kansas City, Missouri: Camp Fire, Inc.
Generations United. 1990. Brochure published by Generations United, c/o
    Child Welfare League of America, Inc., Washington, D.C.
Handbook For Instruction on Aging.   1978.   California State Department of
    Education, Sacramento.
Hauwiller, J., and Jennings, R. 1981. "Counteracting Age Stereotyping With
    Young School Children." *Educational Gerontology* 7:183-190.
Hauwiller, J., R. Jennings, and G. Refsland.   1978.   *Helping Children
    Understand Aging Processes: Gerontology in the Elementary
    Classroom*. Bozeman, Mont.: Montana State University.
John, M.   1977. "Teaching Children about Older Family Members." *Social
    Education* 41:524-27.
Jones, C. 1986. "Grandparents Read to Special Preschoolers." *Teaching
    Exceptional Children*. 19:36-37.
Justiss, A. 1990. Unpublished request for proposal. Tampa, Florida.

Kenny, J. 1988. "Student Community Project in Pittsburgh, Pennsylvania." ACTION, Washington, D.C., VISTA and Student Community Service Programs. Mimeograph.

Lauzon, L. 1981. "Art Project Spans the Generations." *Design for Arts in Education* 83:41-42.

Lyons, C. 1986. "Interagency Alliances Link Young and Old." *Children Today* 15:21-23.

Metal-Corbin, J., D. Corbin, and B. Baker. 1986. "Age Doesn't Matter: Weaving Dance into a Fifth Grade Curriculum." Portions of paper presented at the National AAHPERD Conference in Cincinnati, Ohio, April 13.

Miller, M. 1986. "Elderly Persons as Intergenerational Child Care Providers." *Journal of Employment Counseling* 23:156-61.

Morris, J. 1984. "Project Teen-ager - A Skills Exchange Program: High School Students Volunteering with the Elderly in a Rural Community." Paper presented at the National/International Institute on Social Work in Rural Areas 9th Institute, Orono, Maine, July 28-31.

Orlock, J., and R. Cornish. 1976. *Short Plays For the Long Living*. Boston: Baker's Plays.

Powell, J., and G. Arquitt. 1978. "Getting the Generations Back Together: A Rationale for Development of Community Based Intergenerational Interaction Programs." *The Family Coordinator* 27:421-26.

Ralston, P., et al. 1986. "Enhancing Intergenerational Contact." Curriculum Guide, Iowa State Department of Public Instruction, Des Moines.

Smith, C., and Z. Slinkman. 1982. "Generations Together" MF-651. Cooperative Extension Service, Kansas State University, Manhattan, Kansas.

Smith, C., and G. Gutsch. 1985. "Grandletters" MF752, "Program Instructions" MF 752a, "Grandparent Letters" MF 752b, and "Grandchild Letters." Cooperative Extension Service, Kansas State University, Manhattan, March.

Sorgman, M., M. Sorenson, and M. Johnston. 1979. "What Sounds Do I Make When I'm Old? A Hands-On Approach to Ageism." *Social Education* 43:135-39.

Struntz, K., ed. 1985. *Growing Together: An Intergenerational Sourcebook*. Washington, D.C.: American Association of Retired Persons.

Ventura-Merkel, C. and L. Lidoff. 1983. *Community Planning for Intergenerational Programming*, Volume 8. Washington, D.C.: National Council on the Aging.

"Young and Old Together: A Resource Directory of Intergenerational
        Programs."   1985. California State Department of Education,
        Sacramento.

3
Fundraising

In examining the background histories of the projects discussed in Chapter 2, we may find a number of funding sources from which we can gain data. Project MAIN (Blake 1986) was funded by grants and private foundations, while Channel One (Allen 1986) was provided with seed money from the National Institute on Drug Abuse and support from a Prudential Life Insurance Company manager who identified appropriate communities for the project. A Grandparent Program in California ("Young and Old Together" 1985) was funded through its PTA Advisory Council. Funding for the "Handbook for Instruction on Aging" (1978) came from provisions from the Older Americans Act, Title III, Section 308.

The advantage to cooperative projects between agencies extends to increased funding possibilities. When the program "Developing Intergenerational Programs Jointly with the Aging and Child Care Networks in Pennsylvania" (C. Lyons 1986) was conceived by Generations Together at the University of Pittsburgh Center for Social and Urban Research, funding was obtained from the Administration for Children, Youth and Families and the Administration on Aging.

The Grandparent Read to Me Project (Jones 1986) received a grant in the amount of $2,300 from the Martha Holden Jennings Foundation of Cleveland, Ohio. The SCOPE (Senior Citizen Opportunities in Public Education) project (Firman and Stowell 1980) involved senior citizens as tutors in the San Diego school system. This particular project was funded through the local Area Agency on Aging, under Title V of the Older Americans Act. The Montana intergenerational project, "Providing Gerontological Concepts in the Elementary Classroom: Helping Children Understand the Aging Process" (Hauwiller and Jennings 1981), was supported by a grant from the

Aging Services Bureau, Department of Social and Rehabilitation Services, State of Montana.

Project STEP (Seniors Tutor for Educational Progress) (R. Drummond et al. 1975) offers to interested parties information on budgetary procedures that are "adoptable or adaptable" to other interested school districts.

In 1979, as Director of the Intergenerational Theatre Company, I needed funding to enable the company to travel to schools, agencies, and universities to present oral-history theatre scripts. We were fortunate to receive funding through the Life Insurance Company of Virginia.

Funding sources may be as varied as the projects. It is to the advantage of the project organizers to research available funding sources at local, state, and national levels. As the previous information suggests, there are numerous possibilities; one must match the objective, outcome, and focus of the project with an appropriate funding source, whose purpose it is to support this type of endeavor. Universities have often employed a grants writer or researcher, usually in the development office. Working with local colleges and universities to research possible sources of funding is a natural beginning. Another direction might be local agencies on aging and arts agencies. Both interest groups are community-minded and may be receptive to innovative ideas that promote intergenerational experiences in the arts. A third possible source is local parent-teacher groups, who are usually very supportive of the expansion of educational opportunities and helpful in fundraising and supplying other assistance.

Businesses offer invaluable assistance to various educational projects across the nation and have a vested interest in the success of education in this country. As David Kearnes, the CEO of the Xerox Corporation, and Denis Doyle, Senior Research Fellow at the Hudson Institute, appropriately pointed out recently, "Our schools must teach a love of democracy, and insure that that love is passed on from generation to generation" (D. Kearnes and D. Doyle 1988, p. 142). Quality education was important enough to this business leader and researcher that they devoted an entire book to the topic.

Marvin Cetron, Barbara Soriano, and Margaret Gale (1985, p. 85) further support the relationship between business and school, saying, "While business cooperation with schools is not new, partnerships between businesses and schools will be a pervasive part of the daily operations in most school districts by the 21st century." They further predict that schools of the twenty-first century will be expected to provide learning experiences not only for children but also for students aged from 21 to 80-plus. According to their predictions, it seems plausible that certain businesses with insights into successful futures would be interested in discussing projects now in the developmental stages of planning or implementation.

Three books should also be studied in the preparation of grant proposals: *The Art of Winning Corporate Grants* (H. Hillman and M. Chamberlain, *The Art of Winning Foundation Grants* (H. Hillman and K. Abarbanel 1975), and *The Art of Winning Government Grants* (H. Hillman and K. Natale 1977). These invaluable texts include clearly outlined steps in research and writing and other information applicable to those in need of project support.

MULTIGENERATIONAL-INTEREST GRANTWRITING

An excellent activity to be shared by parents, senior citizens, representatives from agencies, and students from middle or high schools would be cooperative planning and grantwriting for intergenerational programming. Although group writing is often difficult, it can be rewarding if approached in an organized fashion, whereby each group member has input and a task assignment. It is advisable to elect a head writer or perhaps two writers who will be responsible for the final document.

Groups working together will find that the process of brainstorming is perhaps the most effective way to involve all parties and allow for generating creative solutions to problems. All too often programs are planned for teenagers, youth, and senior citizens without their consultation or input. A program designed by, for, and about a particular intergenerational group would yield benefits far greater than passive noninvolvement.

The following guidelines are offered as a way to begin the grantwriting and funding research process:

1. Needs Assessment. Identify the needs of each of the groups. Mix the groups, however. For example, a high school student, a parent representative, a senior citizen, and an agency member would make a strong intergenerational, multi-interest group of people who could help each other to brainstorm effective ideas for implementation.

2. Service and Talent Exchange. After deciding upon the individual needs of each interest group, the next step is to brainstorm ways in which individuals in the group may help each other and exchange services and talents.

3. Goals. An exchange list citing the goals of the project should be drawn up. The group may then try to match these goals with the interests of a funding source or sources. In finding a funding source one must study the goals of the particular source to see if the ideas of the intergenerational group match.

4. Writing. Once research has been conducted and sources identified, the actual writing of the grant may be implemented by the group. Again, group members may work in teams with specific tasks to accomplish such as the introduction to the project, the explanation of the goals, the budget, and plans for implementation.

Having several people work on a grant proposal increases the likelihood of support from each agency and expands the possibility of reaching and affecting the lives of a greater population. When program participants are allowed to plan and design the project, each agency has a vested interest in the outcome, having devoted time to the planning and writing of the project. Furthermore, each organization may have community outreach capabilities that other members of the team may not be aware of. This information may surface through shared discussion and, consequently, the overall knowledge as to the impact of the project will be enhanced.

The actual writing of the grant will be a useful language arts lesson for students of middle and high school levels as the language must be clear, succinct, and well organized and must at the same time appeal to the reader. Students of math may find the budget an exciting challenge because they are also involved in the design of what items will be needed for the project and other expenditures they might incur. Grantwriting and project planning allow students to become involved in an activity that will have an impact upon their present lives and future experiences. The preparation of a grant proposal and budget for a project in which the students will participate makes the writing and studying relevant to the student in the present day.

Participation gives the senior citizens an opportunity to assist in the design of a project that will enhance their lives. It also enables them to continue to contribute to the ongoing process of community involvement, from which seniors are all too often removed because of retirement, segregation, and confinement. Just because one is physically confined, one need not be mentally confined.

Furthermore, as part of the educational intergenerational process, meetings might be held at different locations so that representatives from each group would have the opportunity to visit and work in the environments of the others. Working in the high school library can be a very different experience from working in an agency office. Working in the dining hall or community room of a nursing home can yield insights for all involved and cut through the image of visiting the nursing home only once every two months to sing, play cards, or talk. That is not to say that such visitation projects by various groups are not helpful. On the contrary, they add to the overall well-being and understanding of everyone involved. But when one works in a particular place, rather than visits, the environment of that facility takes on a completely new meaning.

Allowing individuals to have an input into a project also gives them a vested interest. They have firsthand knowledge and can become enthusiastic leaders, thus generating excitement in the community, at school, in the nursing home, and at the agency. The project then becomes true to its original intention for intergenerational socialization and understanding, whether it be a project about tutoring, writing, dance, drama, or shopping for supplies. From its inception it has remained true to the overall goal of getting the generations back together for the betterment of individuals and the community. The nursing home, the agency, and the learning institution then become integral parts of the development, incorporation, and problem-solving processes of multigenerational socialization.

REFERENCES

Allen, M. 1986. "Channel One: An Intergenerational Program at Work." *Children Today* (May - June) 15:32 - 34.

Blake, Gerald. 1986. "Project MAIN: Classwork in the Community Benefits Senior Citizens." *Children Today* (July - August) 15:31 - 34.

Cetron, M., with B. Soriano and M. Gale. 1985. *Schools of the Future: How American Business and Education Can Cooperate to Save Our Schools*. New York: McGraw-Hill Book Company.

Drummond, R., et al. 1975. "Project STEP (Seniors Tutor for Educational Progress)." On-Site Validation Report, Easton-Redding Regional School District 9, Connecticut.

Firman, J., and A. Stowell. 1980. "Intergenerational School Projects: Examples and Guidelines." *Media and Methods* (February):19,42.

"Handbook for Instruction on Aging in California Public Schools." 1978. California State Department of Education, Sacramento.

Hauwiller, J., and R. Jennings. 1981. "Counteracting Age Stereotyping with Young School Children." *Educational Gerontology* 7:183 -90.

Hillman, H. and K. Abarbanel. 1975. *The Art of Winning Foundation Grants*. New York: Vanguard Press.

Hillman, H., and M. Chamberlain. 1980. *The Art of Winning Corporate Grants*. New York: Vanguard Press.

Hillman, H. and K. Natale. 1977. *The Art of Winning Government Grants*. New York: Vanguard Press.

Jones, C. 1986. "Grandparents Read to Special Preschoolers." *Teaching Exceptional Children* 19:36 - 37.

Kearns, D., and D. Doyle. 1988. *Winning the Brain Race*. San Francisco: Institute for Contemporary Studies.

Lyons, C. 1986. "Interagency Alliances Link Young and Old." *Children Today* 15:21 - 23.

"Young and Old Together: A Resource Directory of Intergenerational Programs." 1985. California State Department of Education, Sacramento.

4
Educating the Masses

The complexity of current educational curricula remains one of the most challenging aspects of American society today. While traditionalists fight for "back to the basics" victory, nontraditionalists continue to vie for equal time in the struggle for individual development.

"The notion that a common background knowledge exists is the rational behind the development of any school curriculum. Controversy has always surrounded the building of core curricula, since few people can agree on what that common knowledge should be. The 1980s have seen a backlash against decisions made in the 1960s to integrate new concepts into curricula at the expense of old ideas. The problem, of course, is that world knowledge is not stable; it expands at one end faster than it contracts at the other" (D. Zahler and K. Zahler 1988, p. ix).

One universal force that has the capability of worldwide shared knowledge and understanding is that of the process of aging. Every country has elderly people, and although the inclusion of gerontological studies in public and private education is growing, there remains a need for an overall national/international focus. This knowledge about the aging process is essential to a clearer vision and understanding of the process of living.

"I can't stand going to the nursing home. It's so depressing." This statement came from one of my high school theatre students as we discussed possible trips to the nursing home to perform oral history scripts. This particular student had experiences through the school service club of visiting the nursing home during holidays to deliver fruit baskets. Although this young man was a hard worker and usually open to meeting and working with new people, his previous experiences in the long-term care setting had clouded his youthful dreams of discovery.

Interaction between generations may be affected by perceived physical appearances. Vicki Freimuth and Kathleen Jamieson discuss the concept of homophily in stating that "the more similar two communicators are the more likely it is that they will interact and that their interaction will be successful. One of our first perceptions of homophily is based on appearance" (1979, p .3). With the stress placed on "youthful appearance" in today's advertising, the physical appearance of a seventeen-year-old, compared to that of a seventy-five-year-old, may place an immediate barrier between the two unless there are other common points of reference.

The research is contradictory concerning adolescents' attitudes toward the aging. Connie Ivester and Karl King (1977) found that the attitudes of adolescents in a rural area were more positive toward the elderly than those indicated in earlier studies, during the 1950s and 1960s. A part of this differentiation was attributed to the former studies having been conducted in predominantly urban areas. Another contributing factor to the discrepancy may be the increasing public awareness in the past twenty years of the aged as individuals. One important finding, however, was that frequency of contact with the elderly had a positive effect on the adolescents' views of aging. Although my particular situation involved the reactions of only one student, it must be stated that this did take place in a predominantly rural community.

It is increasingly apparent that not only the quantity but also the quality of contact between the generations is of utmost importance. The moments shared by youth and elderly are vital to the building of understanding and trust, but these may be achieved only through consistently active contact rather than limited nonparticipatory visitation as experienced by this adolescent student.

Negative reactions to the aging process have also been found at the elementary and preschool levels (R. Jantz, C. Seefeldt, A. Galper, and K. Serlock, 1977). However, with the success of such intergenerational programs as previously discussed, these attitudes and stereotypical views are beginning to change. With the success of such pre-training programs as that of Dellman-Jenkins et al. (1986), negative attitudes can be changed through positive interaction. Children may begin to study rather than judge. This is why incorporation of the arts in program planning is so vitally important as artists are asked to investigate, explore, and study subjects rather than pass judgment.

One important component of intergenerational sharing is the pre-training of both parties. Adolescents and children should be given information before they go to the nursing home to ensure adequate preparation, thus avoiding unnecessary shock or depression by initial exposure to various dehabilitating circumstances. Students should be made aware that physical confinement may not necessarily mean intellectual confinement.

EDUCATING THE MASSES THROUGH PUBLIC EDUCATION

The most obvious place to begin educating the masses is through the public school system. In an investigation of curriculum studies in Ohio, Jill Frymier Russell (1979) found that although measurable efforts were being made to teach courses on aging in schools, in many cases these studies were not being offered for three primary reasons: (1) nontraditional topic, (2) lack of adequate materials, and (3) unpreparedness. Russell offers realistic solutions to all three problems, beginning with a course in aging in the teacher-training curriculum. Efforts to include units within the traditional curriculum have been successfully implemented, demonstrating that lessons in aging may not be so nontraditional as originally thought. Russell also suggests in-service training for interested teachers who may want to include this area of study in their regular curricula.

Because the topic of lifelong learning and development encompasses such a wide area of experience, lessons have been developed in almost every traditional subject area. It is especially the arts, however, that offer an expressive avenue through which young and old may work together.

PRE-PROJECT TRAINING - SIMULATED ACTIVITIES

Wheelchair Confinement

Probably one of the most predominant misconceptions held by youth is that those who are confined to wheelchairs are also mentally impaired. To those who are unaccustomed to wheelchairs, the apparatus presents an immediate barrier. The appearance of cold steel may, to the inexperienced participant, present a negative visual barrier. For adolescents the mere proximity of distance between the person sitting and the person standing up presents a physical barrier in communication.

Younger children are less likely to have seen a wheelchair; consequently, the introduction of this apparatus is very important. If children at an early age visit a nursing home, a wheelchair may seem a large piece of frightening machinery with which they are unfamiliar, and apprehension and fear may follow. An excellent series, "Kids on the Block," (S. Nelton 1986) introduces children, through the use of puppets, to various handicapping conditions in a positive way. After the introduction of the puppets a child's wheelchair may be produced, so that children can touch and possibly talk about it. After the introduction of this apparatus, a trip to the nursing home, where some residents may be confined to wheelchairs, becomes a natural experience rather than a frightening ordeal.

Yet another consideration is that, for small children, the proximity of someone seated may work as a positive component. On a similar note, the adolescent may be forced to pull up a chair in order to communicate, thus establishing a more relaxed atmosphere. Yet, without previous experience, students may still find themselves put off by the steel confinement. Using drama sequences as a pre-training activity to role play simulated activities might help the students to better understand this special condition.

Character Chair - A Pre-Training
Simulation Activity

1. Set-up. Ask for the loan of a wheelchair from either an agency or a nursing home. Place the wheelchair in a central part of the classroom where all the students can see it. In the seat of the wheelchair place a card that has written on it:

IF YOU HAD TO SIT IN THIS CHAIR ALL THE TIME WHAT THINGS COULDN'T YOU DO THAT YOU ORDINARILY DO NOW? WHAT THINGS COULD YOU DO THAT WOULD BE DIFFERENT FROM WHAT YOUR FRIENDS COULD DO?

2. Master List. After students have had the opportunity to respond either in writing or through class discussion, compile a master list of COULD DOs and COULDN'T DOs and post it on the wall or board.

3. Simulated Character Observation. Ask for a volunteer to sit in the chair and pretend to be old. The teacher should assign the task of character observer to two other students. They will keep a log of responses, body language, and reactions of other students to the wheelchair-confined participant. Two other students should record the actions and oral responses of the wheelchair participant.

4. Character Sketch. Give the wheelchair participant a card on which has been written his or her age, reason for confinement, and general background information such as place of birth, former occupation, number of children, and favorite hobby.

5. Class Roles. Assign various roles to students in the class, such as "misinformed," who treats the wheelchair participant as if he or she were mentally incapable of answering any questions, making any decisions, or contributing to the group.

6. Alienation. The remainder of the students in the class should each ask the wheelchair- confined person at least one question. At some point during the interviewing process another student who has been assigned the task of "mover" should roll the student away from the group. At another time, the "mover" should roll the student so that his back is to the group. Other techniques such as limiting mobility by tying the hands down, limiting hearing by putting on earmuffs, and limiting sight by placing "play glasses" that have been frosted over on the wheelchair participant may also help to simulate various special circumstances with which students may come into contact.

7. Shared Observation. After students have completed the interviewing process, the teacher should ask the character observers and the wheelchair observer for their observations. The teacher should ask the wheelchair participant for his reactions or observations.

8. Concluding List. The teacher may then, with the help of the students, design a master list of safety and consideration tips for working with wheelchair participants. Some of these tips might include (1) asking or telling the person where he or she is going before you begin to roll the wheelchair. Avoid startling the person. (2) Be aware of where the person is located in relation to a group activity. Can the person hear? Can the

person see? Is he or she sitting next to someone who might cause a problem? (3) If engaged in movement or dance activities, is the person securely placed in the wheelchair to avoid falling? (4) Does the staff prefer that the brakes are left on or off during participation in the activity?

9. Follow-up.   Invite a professional from the community from an agency, university, or nursing home to talk about various diseases, wheelchair or bed confinement, and the aging process. This may be done on the same day, or it may be a follow-up activity.

A variation on this technique may be used for simulating activities for bedridden patients in which a student may be asked to sit outside the classroom or in some isolated area of the room.

INTERCURRICULUM INVOLVEMENT

An intercurriculum class period is possible, with science, psychology, and physical education classes taking part. Each teacher's wide range of knowledge-based ideas would contribute greatly to the learning at hand. The class might elect a person to experience being wheelchair bound for a day at school. Discussion of the difficulties and experiences would certainly benefit all involved.

History and social studies classes may want to make a study of President Franklin D. Roosevelt and all he was able to accomplish from a wheelchair; math classes may want to calculate wheelchair races and/or various Rock-a-thons and wheel-a-thons at nursing homes. Language arts classes could respond through expressive or creative essays about wheelchair experiences. Art and shop classes might design and display their versions of the ULTIMATE wheelchair, the wheelchair of the future.

AWARENESS TRAINING THROUGH LITERATURE

Literature is another approach to motivating discussion and investigation of the aging process in a positive way. For high school students such stories as "The Good Deed" by Pearl S. Buck are excellent for capturing the essence of intergenerational questions concerning values, change, and customs. This particular story concerns the immigration of old Mrs. Pan to America and her subsequent adjustment to the "new customs" of youth, dating, and marriage. An opening question for writing or discussion might be, "If your parents arranged a marriage for you what would your husband or wife be like? Would you agree or disagree with their choice, and why?"

Another language arts activity is the assignment of the topic "How I Feel about Old People." Some of the responses from freshman high school English classes in Chesterfield, Virginia, were as follows: "It's hard to believe some of the things they tell you they did when they were a teenager." "I love them but they scare me bad. I guess because one day I know I'll be like them." "When I get old I want to be just like my grandpaw. He is old and very smart and he can make anyone laugh." "They teach you things that books cannot touch." "I'm going to take my grandkids camping and fishing and teach them how to have fun. I'll try to share my knowledge with them" (Student papers 1988).

Some students went on to describe what they felt they would look like in their elderly years: "I will probably have lots of wrinkles and very little hair and a big long grey beard that took me many years to grow," and "When I get old I'm going to be fat and gray-haired. I'm gonna be fat because I eat a lot of food now and I'll probably be real fat by the time I get old!"

Simulated activities for kindergarten through grade three may begin with story reading as demonstrated by earlier projects. A suggested list of reading materials can be found in the annotated bibliography of this book. Younger children may draw pictures of their grandparents or engage in discussions about grandparents.

One book that particularly stimulates conversation about the elderly is *Kevin's Grandma* by Barbara Williams (1975). Children may be asked to decide what kind of grandmother(s) they have in their family, old-fashioned or modern. It may be helpful, however, first to identify the difference or their perceptions of "old-fashioned" and "modern." Making lists for each category also provides a visual stimulus for discussion. For preschool children, drawing pictures of their grandparents may be substituted for listing words.

PREPARATION AT THE NURSING HOME

The younger participants are not the only persons who should receive pre-training information and experience through simulated activities. It is just as important to dispel stereotypes of youth. Nursing home activity personnel may begin with a discussion of "What is youth?" This may lead to a list of stereotypes concerning younger people. Discussions might also be held concerning the residents' experiences as young children and adolescents. Some helpful subtopics might include the following:

.Changes in values
.Changes in economics
.Changes in customs
.Changes in dress
.Changes in recreation
.Changes in education
.Changes in the family unit
.Changes in discipline

Using resources in the community such as teachers, social workers, and parents to speak with residents about the special needs of children in today's world would also provide helpful pre-project exposure to youth.

A guest speaker may use the list generated earlier through discussion and elaborate upon selected ideas or thoughts concerning the elderly's views of youth. The objective is to dispel myths of youth and at the same time bring the generations closer together through shared interests. Vicki Freimuth and Kathleen Jamieson attest to the importance of understanding others, saying, "The process of forming impressions and making judgments about others is called interpersonal perception. Our deficient interpersonal perception of persons of another generation can result in a breakdown in communication with them" (1979, p.2).

Understanding and communication are of course best accomplished through the final stage of positive interaction between the two groups. The success of positive group interaction, however, may be dependent upon positive training activities and learning.

HELPFUL CONTACTS

Statewide Intergenerational Programs (provided by the National Council on the Aging, 1990)

Illinois Network: Emeritus College
Southern Illinois University
Carbondale, IL 62901
618/536-7735

New Jersey Network: New Jersey Division on Aging
363 West State Street, CN807
Trenton, NJ 08625-0807
609/292-3765

Northern California Intergenerational Program Network:
4032 Maher Street
Napa, CA 94558
707/255-5430

Southern California Intergenerational Program Network: Center for
Community Education
Office of Los Angeles County Superintendent
9300 East Imperial Highway
Downey, CA

Delvin-Delaware Valley Intergenerational Network: Center for
Intergenerational Learning
Temple University
1601 West Broad Street
Philadelphia, PA 19122
215/787-6970

Massachusetts Intergenerational Network:
Old Sturbridge Village
Museum Education Center
Sturbridge, MA 01566

New Mexico Intergenerational Network:
New Mexico Conference of Churches
235 Mezcal Circle, N.W.
Alburquerque, NM 87105

Wisconsin Intergenerational Network:
RSVP
540 West Olin Avenue, #136
Madison, WI 53715
806/256-5596

REFERENCES

Buck, P. "The Good Deed." 1953. In *Understanding Literature* 1984. New
        York: Macmillan.
Dellmann-Jenkins, M., D. Lambert, D. Fruit, and T. Dinero. 1986. "Old and
        Young Together: Effect of an Educational Program on

Preschoolers' Attitudes toward Older People." *Childhood Education* 62:206 -8, 210 - 12.

Freimuth, V., and K. Jamieson. 1979. *Communicating with the Elderly: Shattering Stereotypes*. Urbana, Ill.: ERIC Clearinghouse on Reading and Communication Skills.

Ivester, C., and K. King. 1977. "Attitudes of Adolescents toward the Aged." *The Gerontologist* 17:85 - 90.

Jantz, R., C. Seefeldt, A. Galper, and K. Serlock. 1977. "Children's Attitudes Toward the Elderly." *Social Education* 41:518 -23.

Nelton, S. 1986. "Puppets Promote Understanding." *Nation's Business* 74:70.

Russell, J. "Aging in the Public Schools." 1979. *Educational Gerontology: An International Quarterly* 4:19-24.

Student papers. 1988. Thomas Dale High School, Chesterfield, Virginia.

Williams, Barbara. 1975. *Kevin's Grandma*. New York: E.P. Dutton.

Zahler, D., and K. Zahler. 1988. *Test Your Cultural Literacy*. New York: ARCO.

5

Intergenerational Activities in Drama, Writing, and Poetry

Drama is a natural activity for all ages. It may take different shapes and forms throughout the various stages of life; however, it is an indigenous activity in which we all participate at one time or another. For the very young child, dramatic play is a necessary experience for growth and development; for the adolescent and maturing youth, role playing is a necessary activity in the rehearsal for life. For the young adult, life itself becomes a drama as one is required to react and respond to numerous characters throughout a lifespan. Role playing is a common point of reference among all generations, yet identification of participation throughout a lifespan filled with drama may not be immediately recognized. Once it is studied, however, one begins to recognize several stages of involvement. The first stage of personal dramatic development is dramatic play, which may or may not be a fond memory for adults.

Virginia Koste refers to dramatic play as "any play involving the mental act of imaginative transformation" (1978, p.6). Through dramatic play the young child is able to invent situations, consider responses, and create characters. Dramatic play usually involves relaxation as a component because those involved are freed of daily concerns and pressures and are unaware of their surroundings or interruptions. For the young child, dramatic play is a necessary step in creative development that may also involve language and motor skills. The child is allowed to explore and develop skills without "performing" for an audience or achieving for a critic.

The combination of adults and young children involved in dramatic play activities is an excellent avenue for intergenerational involvement. Although the ability of the adult to become engaged in dramatic play is often hampered by social constraints, one need only observe a mother or father around a toddler to witness a quick reminiscence of what it was like to be young and simply to play.

One approach to involving the generations in dramatic play is through puppet theatre. One must keep in mind that puppets allow the participant to have an actual physical extension, thus reducing the risk of failure. Through this added dimension, which acts as a spokesperson for the manipulator, feelings, ideas, and creative explorations can be expressed that might otherwise be suppressed. If there is failure in some way, the puppet can always take the blame.

Pat Fiske, director of a puppet project for senior citizens attests to the benefits of this type of activity for older persons in stating that, "through their involvement, seniors were able to overcome the effects of physical disabilities and even emotional difficulties they were experiencing. There could be no doubt that their creative potential was still vibrant and that new types of expressive skills could be learned" (1980, p. 21).

INTERGENERATIONAL PUPPET THEATRE

One may make a number of types of puppets, from sock puppets to sophisticated marionettes. For the purpose of budget and possibly time we will discuss the use of scrap materials and paperbag puppets that residents and children may decorate together. An intergenerational exchange might be to have the young children decorate their paper bags as old persons, and the residents of the nursing home decorate their paper bags as young persons. If the program involves very young children, the seniors may work with them and help to decorate a puppet together.

Paperbag Puppet Show

Suggested materials: paper lunch bags, construction paper, ribbons, scrap fabric, glue, "found" supplies as decorations, crayons, markers, stick-on stars, safety scissors

Supplies appropriate for the abilities of the ages and skills should be gathered by the teacher and activities assistants.

Instructions:

1. Partner Assignment. Assign "Puppet-Partners." Each older resident will receive a young partner to work with.

2. Decoration/Puppet Introduction. Allow residents and children to work together to decorate their puppets. Give participants a specified amount of time to work. Teacher and aides should circulate to assist wherever needed.

If the residents and children have made separate puppets, call for time and have them engage in dramatic play. Call this "get to know your puppet partner," where partners introduce their puppets to the other. The teacher should give verbal encouragement such as "Find out how old your puppet partner is," and "What's your puppet partner's favorite kind of ice cream?"

If the resident and the child have decorated a puppet together, then they will form a "foursome" with another pair and follow the same instructions.

3. Writing Puppet Plays. After engaging in dramatic play, allow groups to write playlets for the puppets. The teacher may want to focus on the intergenerational aspect and ask each group to create a scene concerning an old person and a young person.

For the very young child this will involve oral creativity whereby the story is simply acted out without a script and will more closely resemble dramatic play.

For the older child this may involve writing down a play synopsis and improvising the dialogue or may involve writing lines for each puppet to say.

4. Puppet Theatre Scriptwriting. A suggested title might be "The Little Old Bag Lady" (a formal script is available in the Appendix A). Students may invent a script that centers around an older person or older animal who lives on the street rather than in a house or with a family. The teacher should encourage the groups to include a beginning, middle, and end to the story to assist the group in staying on task.

5. Adaptive Puppet Stages. Mobile puppet stages may be built around a wheelchair by using a piece of cardboard across the front of the chair at a comfortable height for the puppeteers to hold and manage their puppets.

6. Visual Arts Extension. A visual arts extension might be to take photographs of the puppet partner teams with their puppets and to display these pictures at the school and at the nursing home. The title of the play may be written across the top of the display, and a fill-in-the-blank information sheet may be attached. For the nursing home display, the fill-in-the-blank sheet might include the following:

This is my special puppet partner from——————————.
(name of school)

She (he) is————————— years old.

Her puppet's name is ——————————————.

Her puppet's favorite ice cream is ——————————.

My partner's favorite ice cream is ——————————.

The title of our puppet play was ————————————————.

COSTUME PARADE

One of the most enjoyable activities for younger children is that of "dressing up." Costumes may be created from construction paper, sheets, newspapers, scarfs, a variety of hats, and paper plates and cups. In this particular activity, the generations work together as partners to "create" costumes that may center around a theme, focus upon a period in history, or be based upon characters either invented by the group or taken from literature the students have been studying.

The shared costume creation and parade also involve tactile exchange where partners are engaged in touching each other in order to create a costume. Janis Bardi Cardosi addresses two important questions when referring to nursing home residents in asking, "How many of those people die from tactile deprivation and how many more fail to thrive because they have lost this most important physical contact?"(1982, p.3).

Although the beginning stages of costume creation may be categorized as functional-professional for the purpose of accomplishing a task (J. Cardosi, p. 2), the development of the costume may lead to what Cardosi and R. Heslin refer to as the friendship-warmth category, which is an important life encourager for both the elderly and the young.

Costume Creation and Character Parade

Suggested materials: Masking tape, construction paper, newspapers, sheets, towels, old hats, paper plates, cups, crayons, markers, scarfs

Instructions

1. Character Bag. Teacher should have titles of characters in a paper bag which children and elderly persons will draw from. Titles may include king, queen, princess, soldier, magician, dragon, prince, village gossip. (Again, children should work with elderly partners to create costumes for and on each other.)

2. Costume Creation. After each participant has selected a character title, give each group or set of partners a selection of the listed supplies. Allow the participants time to create costumes according to the titles they have drawn from the bag. The teacher/leaders will probably be the best judges of appropriate time limits for their students and residents. (One suggestion is to play soothing music in the background while participants are creating their costumes. A good choice might be Vivaldi, which encourages a synthesis of left and right brains).

3. Costume Parade. Upon the completion of the costumes participants should have a parade through a

designated part of the nursing home to show bed-confined residents their costumes. Participants should then return to the central room (or wherever it is they are working) and bring the parade into a circle.

4. Improvisational Play. At this point, the teacher may guide the participants through an improvisational play about a fantasy land where the elderly save the youth of the kingdom or vice versa. (See Appendix A for outline of the Fantasy Land Play.)

5. Visual Arts/ Writing Extension. Again, as for the paper bag puppet theatre, the group may want to dress in their costumes and have pictures taken for display or for a scrapbook. The teacher and/or group leader may take the scrapbook one step further by having the residents and children write reflective essays concerning their experiences with costuming.

6. Storybook Costume Theatre. With smaller children, the teacher may want to use characters from a book that has been read to the group. One book with animal characters that addresses the intergenerational theme is *It's So Nice to Have a Wolf around the House* (H. Allard 1977).

STORYBOOK THEATRE

The costume parade provides a natural progression into storybook theatre, a technique where residents and children may either create a story and act it out or act out a story based upon a book. One excellent intergenerational book is *Emma* (Kesselman 1980). This particular book allows children to investigate a sense of family through the examination of how older persons are treated by younger family members. Opportunities for creative visual arts are also a consideration as the main character in the book, Emma, discovers her artistic talents. A scripted version of this children's story may be found in the book *Seniors on Stage* (P. Clark and N. Osgood 1985, pp. 137-42).

A second book that focuses on the intergenerational theme is *Miss Rumphius* (Cooney 1982). In this particular story, we follow Miss Rumphius in her journey around the world, thus allowing students also to study geography. One excellent point is made through the grandfather at the beginning of the story and reiterated by Miss Rumphius at the end of the story. Each offers the following advice to a young person, "You must do something to make the world more beautiful."

After sharing the book with the group the teacher may ask the participants what it is they could do to make the world more beautiful and have them act it out. For example, giving a hug to each person in the room would make the world more beautiful, and participants might actually do this. Discovering a cure for a particular disease might be acted out. Students could invent a scene showing research scientists either looking for a cure or making a discovery.

Discussion that offers students an insight into what it means to make the world more beautiful may precede this exercise. In the story Miss Rumphius planted flowers, but participants should be asked if the deed must be visible in order to be effective. This exercise and book are also excellent catalysts for reassuring the elderly that they still have the capability of making a contribution to the world.

A third intergenerational text is *A Treasure Hunt* (Wilson 1980). In this story elderly people in a neighborhood are concerned about the values of the young people. In an effort to bring the generations closer together, they set up a treasure hunt. Each item the children find in the treasure hunt brings them to a better understanding of the elderly in the neighborhood. The discovery of each item also teaches them a skill through the help of the elderly. After this book is read to the group, each child might find out either what their elderly partner did for a living or a special skill or hobby the partner possesses. The child, in turn, shares this information with the other participants. The group may then elect to act out the story, using the skills of the elderly in the room. For example, if one resident was a carpenter by trade, he (she) might set up a pretend carpentry shop where children watch as he mimes carpentry. If possible a follow-up session with some of the residents actually sharing their trades and hobbies would be very effective in actually carrying out the essence of the book.

The activities discussed up to this point involve improvisational theatre and creative dramatics techniques recommended for the primary grades, one through four. The middle and high schools may use the same techniques of creative drama and improvisational theatre but may also feel a need to work on a more structured project that involves writing, researching, and more-formalized production techniques.

LIVING NEWSPAPER PROJECT

The living newspaper project which combines research, writing, and dramatic skills, has been successfully used by middle and high school students in intergenerational settings to explore history and to write dramatic scripts based upon research. As forerunner of the television docudrama, the living newspaper has its roots in the Works Progress Administration's Federal Theatre Project of the 1930s. Elmer Rice provides the following description of the Living Newspaper:

> At first it was planned to present dramatizations of current news events, but it soon became evident that the news would be stale by the time shows could be written and staged. It was then decided to use background material of a more or less topical nature, and scripts were prepared by newswriters dealing with the Ethiopian crisis, the agricultural situation brought about by the depression, and the slum problem. The last named was called *One-Third of A Nation*, a phrase borrowed from President Roosevelt's statement to the effect that one-third of the nation was ill-fed, ill-housed and ill-clothed. These productions employed a fluid, cinematographic technique and were lively and exciting (1959, p.159).

The elderly offer excellent research resources as students may call upon them for interviews concerning the progress of transportation, women's rights, politics, the stock market crash, the Depression, and any number of historical moments they have lived through. Because the living newspaper entails not only reference research but interviews as well, students are also afforded the opportunity to practice communication skills. The elderly, in turn, are given the occasion to reminisce and contribute in a worthwhile way to the education of the youngsters. The textbooks and reference materials are thus enhanced by colorful, firsthand recollections of these important years in history.

The teacher and activities personnel may want first to study this period of theatre history and, more specifically, the Living Newspaper. Some excellent scripts for review are *Injunction Granted*, produced in 1936, which explored the history of labor in the courts; *Created Equal*, an exciting investigation of the principles of freedom and equality in America; and *Triple-A Plowed Under* (DeRohan 1973), a hauntingly familiar topic concerning agricultural problems brought about by the Depression. In fact, many of the topics addressed by the living newspaper staff in the 1930s are the same problems we as a nation face today; students can study a topic not only from a historical point of view but also from a current perspective.

The script of the living newspaper differs from that of the conventional play in that, before it is written, facts, data, and information are collected by a research team. Through investigation, research, and interviews, pertinent information is collected, compiled, and developed into a living newspaper script. Advice to prospective writers given in a manual entitled *Writing the Living Newspaper*, issued by the Federal Theatre Project in 1937, suggested that the goal should be "to compress and carefully apportion every facet of a socially important topic" and that "authenticity should be the guiding principle." Records also indicate that the following method was used in establishing corroborating sources:

> Therefore, each piece of research submitted by the staff should have, at its heading: the name of the research worker, the date of the assignment, the source of information, i.e., the date of the news article, the periodical, or the title and page of the volume from which it is taken. This basic information is necessary to comply with the principle of authenticity in all scripts -- which incidentally, should be annotated when finished. (p. 4)

In beginning this project a review of literature about the organization of the living newspaper staff is helpful.

Although writing a living newspaper script was generally a collective effort, a coordinator, or city editor, was responsible for properly classifying assignments, regulating the flow of assignments, and seeing that all deadlines were met. The city editor was also responsible for the maintenance of a properly indexed file. A student may be assigned the role of city editor while others act as researchers. Residents in the nursing home may serve as living resources.

The second phase to this project is the writing and subsequent production of the script. (See Appendix B for Living Newspaper forms used in previous intergenerational productions.) It is possible for individual participants at the nursing home and at the school to write the script together. Once all research has been gathered, including reference materials and interviews, the topic may be broken into subtopics and assigned to intergenerational play writing teams.

Living Newspaper Play Writing Teams

The play writing teams should study the collected research and discuss a possible "treatment" for the scene, including characters in the scene, setting, central focus, and message. The original living newspaper techniques also encouraged dance, music, puppetry, and rear projection to enhance selected scenes. Consequently, this project may become a multimedia arts experience for the participants.

A further consideration is whether or not to use a loudspeaker to communicate facts to the audience or to relay information through the dialogue itself. The original living newspaper scripts first used the loudspeaker as an actual commentator who could be located either on or off stage and could interject facts concerning statistics or reports that supported the scene taking place on stage. The loudspeaker might also question the actions of the characters. The original function of the loudspeaker was to introduce characters, dates, and localities, however, it later developed a personality of its own:

> The loudspeaker, unlike the protagonist, plays many roles in the living newspaper. Moreover, it is more removed from the play - no matter how much it is personified, it is still closer to being in a neutral position than is the protagonist....The loudspeaker changes sides too often to allow the audience to completely empathize or sympathize with it. In this way, the loudspeaker keeps the objective viewpoint going, when all other viewpoints - the character's, the protagonist's and the audience's - have become subjective or biased. (D. Bowers, 1976, p. 8)

A final consideration while pulling the entire script together, is whether or not to use the loudspeaker technique as a transitory device between scenes, as the script may cover an extensive span of history.

A final component of the living newspaper project is the typing of the script. Since the original living newspapers also included comprehensive bibliographies and footnotes, the intergenerational script should follow suit. This is an excellent unit for students to study bibliographic and footnoting techniques. A further suggestion is to take pictures of the actual production and include photographs with the script. Scripts may later be bound as a lasting memento of the project.

This project may be as complicated or as simplified as deemed necessary by the teacher and participants. As a technique, the living newspaper was distinguishable for its adaptability to production on various scales ranging from union halls to Madison Square Garden in New York City before an audience of over twenty thousand people. This project may be adapted for either a small audience or for a presentation before the community and families.

Considering the topic is certainly as important an element as is the deciding on a topic for a written research paper. Suggestions for topics in the manual *Writing the Living Newspaper* include "warfare, both actual and imminent, the struggle between progress and reaction, the vicissitudes of politics, the advance of science, the fight for the preservation of civil liberties, labor's organizational activities, and the problems of youth"(p. 7). Topics from the past may correspond to present worldwide considerations, enabling the young student to make a correlation between past and present history.

The living newspaper may become a viable research paper, complete with actors, scenes, costumes, dance, and music, which contributes to both generations an experience of collaborative investigation and creation.

Closely linked to the experience of the living newspaper is that of oral history theatre. While the living newspaper addresses national topics, oral history theatre may reenact a moment of reminiscence in an elderly person's life, thus giving the younger student an opportunity to learn about everyday events in history.

ORAL HISTORY THEATRE

The success of oral history theatre has clearly been demonstrated by several professional theaters around the nation including the Actors Theatre of Louisville and the Guthrie Theatre (P. Clark and N. Osgood 1985). Intergenerational oral history theatre carries the process a step further by combining the memories of the elderly and youth to produce an interwoven script of young and old tales.

The elderly possess a wealth of life stories to be shared with younger generations. It is through these stories that youngsters may learn how to better cope with their current dilemmas and may, furthermore, be surprised to find that some of the problems of adolescents have not changed over the generations.

Intergenerational Oral History Theatre

Supplies: Tape recorder, journals, pens, pencils

Instructions

1. Choice of Topic. The intergenerational group should decide upon various topics to discuss. Some suggestions that lend themselves to shared experiences

are dating customs and how they have changed, transportation including driving a car, changes in education, changes in fashion, and changes in the family unit and discipline.

2. Discussion. The discussion might begin with the adolescents asking questions of their senior adult partners and tape-recording the responses. The senior adults may then interview their younger partners. The tapes should be transcribed and then shared during a large group meeting.

3. Review and Scene Selection. After reviewing the collected stories and reflections, the group should decide upon those stories that lend themselves to scenes that can be acted out.

4. Script Development. Scripts can be developed by using improvisational techniques, that is, allowing actors to develop dialogue as they go along, critiquing the effectiveness of the dialogue, and keeping that which seems to move the scene in a natural progression and/or adding other dialogue or action to support the scene development. Participants may want to suggest definite lines to include in the script and work around these choices of dialogue.

The length of each scene may vary, depending upon the subject. One principle to consider, however, is to keep each scene short enough to hold the attention of the audience, but long enough to adequately cover the topic.

5. Role-reversal. An interesting technique is to use role-reversal, where the younger generation takes on the roles of the senior adults and the seniors take on the roles of the younger people.

6. Generation Interaction. In many cases, the script will call for all participants to act. In these instances, the opportunity for interaction between the generations is at a maximum capacity.

7. Performance; and Follow-up Discussion. Performances may be offered at the nursing home or at the school with follow-up discussion sessions which involve audience members.

The following are examples of intergenerational oral history outlines taken from actual working sessions between adolescents and senior adults in a nursing home (P. Clark 1988).

"School Days-Don't Spare the Ruler Days"

Personal experiences: As a child, a senior adult had been sent to the principal's office for disciplinary reasons. An adolescent was afraid of the principal.

Who: Principal -played by a younger person
Teacher - played by a senior adult
Students - played by remainder of participants

Significant Dialogue: "Sometimes you've got to spank them with your tongue! With what you say!"

"First Date- Out Late"

(Role-Reversal)

Personal experience: A senior adult remembered a first date where she had returned home past curfew. An adolescent had remembered the same experience.

Who: Mother - played by a younger generation participant (Irate - waiting up for daughter)
Daughter - played by a senior adult (returning home late)
Boyfriend - played by a senior adult (sheepishly trying to get a kiss)

Significant dialogue: "I know I'm late but I have a perfectly legitimate reason. Oh, you said that *too*?!"

The impact of intergenerational oral history theatre is impressive. Not only do the actor-participants gain a greater understanding of each other, but audience members, through directed discussion, are also able to benefit from the life experiences of each generation. Production of this type of theatre is also very flexible, as costumes, sets, music, and lighting or any combination thereof may be used while an effective message and lesson is produced for the audience and players alike.

Intergenerational theatre need not be limited to middle and high school students. Successful oral history projects such as the Tiny Hearts and Aged Hands Program at the Hillhaven Rehabilitation and Convalescent Center in Asheville, North Carolina, was implemented with a class of third-graders (Perschbacher 1984). Instead of dramatic production, however, a newspaper containing the oral histories of senior adults written and edited by these youngsters served as the communication link between staff, families, and residents.

RADIO DRAMA PRODUCTION

Up to this point we have discussed the writing of scripts for visual dramatic production. There is yet another form of shared writing that is very effective in an intergenerational setting, that of radio drama. Although this genre of writing may be considered a lost art, it should not be forgotten. The contributions of radio drama are enormous, and most senior adults will fondly recall such shows as "Amos 'n Andy," Will Rogers, Burns and Allen, and "Fibber McGee and Molly" (A. Wertheim 1979). The advantage to this type of writing is that it allows the author or authors to focus on one aspect of sensory composition, that of hearing. In teaching middle and high school writing, students sometimes find the concept of sensory writing overwhelming. How can one focus upon taste, smell, sound, sight, and touch, and still write something that makes sense? With radio drama, students are given the luxury of concentrating on one sensory component.

In sharing this type of writing, the student's reward is doubled, with both a pride in hearing the composition read aloud, and a certain excitement in listening as the various characters come to life. This type of project also offers the opportunity for participation through creating sound effects for people with speech, hearing, and sight impairments. Visual cues may be given to those with hearing and speech impairments while touching signals may be given to those with sight impairments. Because this type of writing requires a fine sensibility directed toward sound, it is necessary to engage in some exploratory activities before the initial writing of the script.

Pre-writing Activities

Throughout all of the sound exercises the teacher or activities leader should encourage "active" listening and use this as a cue term. Remind participants that active listening is listening with the entire body, blocking out anything that might interfere such as thinking about a homework assignment due next period or the next meal. Those with hearing impairments might be encouraged to participate by feeling the vibrations of a particular sound.

First allow writing partners simply to listen to sounds inside the room, outside of the room, and outside of the building. Each team should make a list of the sounds they heard. Lists should then be shared with the entire group. The participants should then proceed to the next activity.

A. Sound Description

> Supplies: Tape recorder; one container with water; one empty container; a supply of various objects that make distinguishable sounds such as a bell, two spoons, and anything else the teacher might find appropriate; pens, pencils, and paper

Instructions

1. Designation of Roles. The teacher or activities leader should designate a team from the group to be the "sound presenters" who will make sounds with the various objects.

Note: For those with hearing loss, special adaptations may be made such as allowing that person to feel the object; for those who have difficulty writing, allow their partners to do the writing.

2. Sound Presentation. Writers and their partners either should be blindfolded or should turn their backs to the "sound presenters." "Sound presenters" then use one of the objects to make the first sound and call "Sound number one!"

3. Responding to Sound #1. The teacher or activities leader should have students respond to the following questions regarding the sound:

a. What do you think the object is?

b. What color do you think it is?

c. Where would this object be located?
   (in what environment?)

4. Responding to Sound #2. "Sound presenters" use the object to make the sound a second time. Be sure to give writers the opportunity to listen carefully.

d. What type of character might use this object?

e. If you were to write a scene based on this sound what type of play would it be? Mystery? Comedy? Tragedy? Why? If the visiting class is a language arts, music, or dance class, the teacher may wish at this point to talk about the "mood" of a story, composition of music or dance.

Note: Team members may discuss reactions with each other and make the writing a collaborative effort.

f. Team members should share their responses with the entire group.

After sensitizing the group to general sounds, the next progression in the creation of actual scripts is to focus on specific environmental sounds.

Found Sounds

Supplies - Notecards; felt-tip markers

Instructions

1. Preparation. Teacher or activities leader should prepare four notecards with the following written on each card: Beach, Country, City, Mountains.

Divide the group members into parties of four or five if possible and have them draw a notecard from a hat. The group members should not tell other groups what is written on their cards.

2. Sound Search. Allow groups to travel anywhere in the room to search for and create "found sounds" using objects in the room and their own voices to recreate a moment that best corresponds with the environment written on their card.

Allow groups to practice their "sound scenes."

3. Active Listening Share. Call all groups back to a central meeting area and place the cards back in the hat. Give groups numbers of order and allow each group to make their presentation. Other participants should close their eyes and listen ACTIVELY.

Allow listening participants to guess the location.

4. Adding Dialogue to Active Listening. After they have correctly guessed the location, have participants close their eyes and listen to the presentation a second time. This time encourage listeners to add dialogue that supports the environment. For example, if we are at the beach, listeners might say, "Hey, let's go in the water. It's too hot!"

Groups may wish to use one of the "sound scenes" as a basis for writing a radio script, or they may generate an entirely new idea for a story. It is advisable to focus upon one scene at a time, or the task becomes overwhelming for those involved.

The actual process of writing may be done in a group of four or five or by twosomes. The makeup of groups should be decided upon according to the needs and talents of those involved. A simple rule: the more people involved in a process, the more complicated the task becomes. However, a group of four or five participants may generate more ideas. It is also possible to assign various tasks such as scriptwriter, sound effects person, cue person, director, actor(s), and musical director.

The activities leader or teacher may want to suggest a theme around which each group writes, such as families, schooldays, exploration, or being trapped. For those who have a difficult time getting started, a fill-in-the-blank radio mystery might be used. In this technique, participants are provided with an outline and may continue the writing process (See Appendix A).

Production

The actual recording of the radio drama is probably the most difficult phase of this exercise, but it is also the most fun. Before recording, the group should rehearse a number of times to make certain everyone understands what the sound cues are and when they should be used. The assignment of someone as director helps tremendously in organizing this project. In working with youngsters, job descriptions should be clearly stated or perhaps even written down. For example:

Director:

1. Calls everyone to attention and focus
2. Begins rehearsals and/or tapings
3. Offers suggestions in a positive way to actors and technical crew
4. Listens to suggestions of other members of the group
5. Thanks the group members for their work

Job descriptions may also be created by group members and voted upon. Many times group work fails simply because participants are not aware of their particular responsibilities. Job descriptions also enable the teacher to give students credit for their work through a checklist system.

Upon the completion of the taping, activities leaders may choose to play the tapes over an intercom system in the nursing home, or school personnel may wish to share the tapes at school. The joy in hearing one's own voice as a character or hearing a sound effect one has been instrumental in creating cannot be measured. Individual self-esteem is heightened as each person makes a contribution to the project. The sense of group effort, working together to create a tangible and meaningful project in an intergenerational setting, is an experience long to be remembered and stored on tape. An added advantage is, of course, the opportunity for both parties to develop their writing skills.

DEVELOPING AND DISCOVERING WRITING SKILLS

Discovering the ""writing voice" within one's self is truly an uplifting experience. For youngsters, it is a source of pride and accomplishment and a renewed sense of success. Positive views of writing are expressed by some adolescents, while others, most of whom have had negative experiences, shy away from this form of self-expression. Adolescents especially need positive avenues of self-expression. The discovery of the ability to write and to communicate feelings and ideas that are appreciated by others provides them with a joyful and rewarding experience.

For the elderly, writing may be a rediscovery of sleeping talents. Having the time to write during the working years is a luxury to most; by retirement age, writing skills may be dormant. Another possibility is that, during the time senior adults attended school, creative writing was not part of the regular curriculum. "Fear of writing" is not only limited to the young or to the elderly. How many times have we heard friends, family or colleagues say, "Boy, I could write a book about that, but I'm a terrible writer!"? *All* ages have a need to express themselves, their stories or ideas. It is through intergenerational writing that both individual and communal discoveries are made.

Some suggested shared writing experiences include the following:

1. Autobiographical Comparisons - Family Trees

2. Family Stories (Sad and Happy)

3. Comparing/Contrasting Reactions to Music, Films, or Ideas

4. The Most Interesting Person in My Family's History

5. Responding to Aphorisms ("A penny saved is a penny earned.") An excellent source is the text *Aphorisms: A Personal Selection* (W.H. Auden and L. Kronenberger 1981), which contains interesting aphorisms pertaining to, among other numerous topics, youth and old age.

6. Creating Aphorisms Together

One type of writing yet to be explored is intergenerational poetry. Two responses I often hear from my students are, "I love to write poetry!" and "I hate poetry!" When asked why they hate poetry, many say, "It's too hard to understand; it's boring," and "I'm not good at writing it. I always get a bad grade." Although it is indeed difficult to find a fair system of grading for poetry, it is possible to evaluate poetry, depending upon the form, or to award points for process rather than product work.

INTERGENERATIONAL POETRY

Writing poetry with someone else alleviates some of this apprehension in that there is a second party who is willing to accept responsibility for creative choices. Working together may also generate ideas that might not otherwise surface. Again, getting started may be the most difficult part for participants. If the students and senior adults have been involved in any of the found-sounds exercises, then intergenerational poetry may be used as an extension of this activity. If, however, there is a need to explore poetry as a separate unit, the following activities may serve as a catalyst for team writing.

Searching for Senses

Students and senior adults should first concentrate on the senses by making a list or the teacher may prepare a list and display it at the front (or somewhere where it is easily visible) of the classroom. Students and senior adult partners should brainstorm responses to the following cues.

1. Hearing (teacher encouragement cues): What kinds of sounds are in the room? How loud are they? How soft are they? Is there a rhythm?

2. Sight (teacher encouragement cues): What is the brightest color in the room? The darkest color? Is there something round? What is it? Something square? What is it? How many people are in the room? What color is the floor? What is the shape of the room?

3. Touch (teacher encouragement cues): What can you reach out and touch without getting up? What does it feel like? If you were able to touch the ceiling what would it feel like? Is there a rough object in the room? What would it be like to touch it? Reach down and touch the floor. What does it feel like? Is it warm? Cold? (Again, safety comes first. If some residents are wheelchair-bound and it is difficult for them to touch the floor, have their partner describe it to them.)

4. Smell (teacher encouragement cues): What do you smell in the room? Is it a good smell? How would you describe it? (This particular sense may be a very delicate matter as sometimes there are unpleasant odors in nursing homes, or a resident may have had physical difficulty. At the same time, an adolescent who has forgotten deodorant might offer the same experience. The teacher or activities leader should use his or her own judgement in using this particular part of the exercise. One alternative might be for the leader to suggest that everyone look outside and imagine what the smells are, or, if weather permits, to actually conduct the class outside.)

5. Taste (teacher encouragement cues): Is there something you taste in your mouth at the moment? How would you describe it?

6. Sixth Sense (teacher encouragement cues): What is the general atmosphere in the room? How do you think people are feeling? Is there a mood or feeling to the room? How would you describe it?

Controlled Search

The participants should go through the same process as in the preceding activity, but the teacher should offer each group or team an actual object such as slices of an apple or lemons or offer various objects to the different groups. (As a preliminary precaution, teachers should check with nurses to see if there are residents with special dietary concerns.) Add controlled sounds such as a particular musical selection, a bell, or party noisemaker. Drape various colored scarfs or sheets across chairs in front of the participants. Pass around a scented candle or a variety of spices. Allow groups to discuss their reactions to the various objects that have been passed around.

The next step is to assign a selection of objects to each group or team. These will become the motivators for their poetry writing. Ask teams to look once again at their objects and decide whether they would like to write descriptions of them or reflections about people who use these objects.

There are several avenues to take in the writing process including free writing (writing without regard to criticism and grading, closely resembling "stream-of-consciousness" flow), pre-writing, outlining, jotting down ideas, and clustering (using visual display and key words while placing the main idea, word, or phrase in the middle of the paper in a box or circle and working by thought association from the central point outward). The selection of direction depends largely upon the teacher and the activity director for both know which methods are most effective with their students and clientele.

Another method that lends itself to intergenerational considerations is the following exercise:

Complete a Thought

Instructions

An intergenerational writing team is given nutmeg, a red scarf, a bell, and a slice of apple. The youngster rings the bell and completes the following thought:

When I ring the bell I hear————
————————————————————————.
(He or she hands the bell to his/her senior adult partner)

When   she   rings   the   bell   she
hears————————————————————.
(Student writes down the reaction of the senior adult)
When   I   see   the   red   scarf   I   think
of————————————————.
When   she   sees   the   red   scarf   she   thinks
of————————————.
When   I   bite   into   the   apple   I
taste————————————————.
When   she   bites   into   the   apple   she
tastes————————————.
When   I   smell   the   nutmeg   I   think
of————————————————.
When   she   smells   the   nutmeg   she   thinks
of————————————.

Depending upon the responses, this exercise may remain a poem unto itself, or the team may want to look at its members' responses and work with them separately to create a new poem. The same method may be used for comparing ages, backgrounds, education, or families. For example:

I am eighty-three,
He is but twelve.
Seventy-one years lies
between the lines in our hands
Yet, in a hug we are
one.

Living Poetry Presentation

In taking poetry one step further, we engage in the combination of creative movement and drama to form a living poetry presentation. The poem becomes a dramatic script as the senior says:

I am eighty-three
(*either steps forward or rolls forward*),

He is but twelve.
(*Youth steps forward*)

Seventy-one years lie
between the lines in our hands
(*Both may use arms and hands in a circular motion or draw hands away from each other.*)

Yet, in a hug
(*Senior adult and youth go towards each other and hold out arms to each other in preparation for a hug.*)

We are
one.
(*Senior adult and youth hug and perhaps hold up fingers to indicate number one.*)

The actual presentations of poetry will naturally depend upon the interpretation and content of the poems. Music, scarfs, backdrops, sound effects, and audience participation can be incorporated into the poetry presentation if the addition enhances the meaning and style of the original poem.

There are, of course, many different types of poetry to explore - haiku, ballad, cinquain, narrative, - and many more which the teacher and activity director may choose to investigate with the residents and youths. Each type of poetry will dictate a particular rhythm that makes this type of dramatic presentation compatible with the exercise.

The study of poetry that addresses the topic of the generations is yet another worthwhile venture. Such poems as "The Old One and the Wind" (Short 1971), "I Miss Being Needed," "Shaving," "Change," and "I Don't Hear as Well as I Used To" (Maclay 1977) are all excellent avenues for reading, pondering, and discussing. In a study of selected poetry listed in *Granger's Index to Poetry* (Smith 1973), M. Sohngen and R. Smith (1978) concluded that "the images of old age found in the most readily available poems are similar to the negative stereotypes of popular culture." As students work in intergenerational settings, their response to these poems and to this particular study would certainly lend itself to interesting discussions of the evolving views of aging.

Another interesting study is that of Martha Clark (1980) in which contemporary American poetry written by artists sixty years of age and older was reviewed. Through this review, Clark responded positively to findings of important key life concepts such as "awareness" and "the passing on of lived experience." Her final statement concerning the study is worth reflection: "that so many of the poems value continued struggle, change, growth, and self-realization in old age leads me to think that there runs, somewhere, a great river of strength among our elders"(1980, p. 191).

DRAMATIC LITERATURE

For those interested in the study and production of actual scripts, there is a wealth of intergenerational dramatic literature available for formal staging. One must keep in mind production costs and royalty fees in producing for a paying public. However, in-class study of selected scenes that address understanding between the generations is certainly a worthwhile educational activity. One play included in the Macmillan literature series *Understanding Literature* (1984), for freshman high school English, is *A Sunny Morning* by Serafin and Joaquin Alvarez Quintero (1920). The level of this one-act appeals to ages fourteen and beyond as it explores a rediscovered love affair between two senior adults. In contrast, we have two young people in the play, one of whom, the female, acts as a subtle shadow in her youthful ventures with life and love. Another interesting aspect of this play is in its approach to presenting the two elderly characters at the beginning of the play as stereotypically "grumpy" and unwilling to change. By the end of the play, however, we know them as individuals.

On Golden Pond (Thompson 1979) offers excellent opportunities for intergenerational scene study as we examine the relationship between a youth and his eighty-year-old future stepgrandfather. Through the acting and discussion of selected scenes from the play, younger participants may better relate to personal experiences with grandparents and the elders may better understand their grandchildren. Communication is, after all, the intent of intergenerational programming, with the hoped-for outcome being a greater shared understanding of the life process.

Dramatic exercises, writing, performances, and interpretation offer endless opportunities for communicating not only between generations but with an audience as well. Thus, the impact reaches far beyond the immediate experience of the participants as productions, readings, writings, and creative endeavors are shared with the community, families, and friends, making the final outcome a joyful celebration of human sharing.

HELPFUL ADDRESS

Institute on the Federal Theatre Project and New Deal Culture
A407 Performing Arts Building
George Mason University
Fairfax, VA 22030-4444

REFERENCES

Allard, H. 1977. *It's So Nice to Have a Wolf around the House*. New York: Doubleday and Company.

Alvarez Quintero, S., and J. Quintero. 1920. "A Sunny Day" In *Understanding Literature*. 1984. New York: Macmillan.

Auden, W.H., L .and Kronenberger. 1981. *Aphorisms*. New York: Penguin Books.

Bowers, D. 1976. "Ethiopia." George Mason University publication.

Cardosi, J. 1982. "I Remember How My Mother Used to Hold Me, God: A Look at Touching the Elderly." Paper presented at the Virginia Speech Communication Association, Rhetoric and Communication Theory Division, October.

Clark, M. 1980. "The Poetry of Aging: Views of Old Age in Contemporary American Poetry." *The Gerontologist* 20:188-91.

Clark, P. 1988. Journal Entries. Lucy Corr Nursing Home, Chesterfield County, Virginia.

Clark, P., and N. Osgood. 1985. *Seniors on Stage: The Impact of Applied Theatre Techniques on the Elderly*. New York: Praeger Publishers.

Cooney, B. 1982. *Miss Rumphius*. New York: Viking Press.

DeRohan, P., ed. 1973. *Federal Theatre Plays*. New York: DeCapo Press.

Heslin, R. 1974. "Steps Toward A Taxomony of Touching." Paper presented at the Midwestern Psychological Association, Chicago.

Kesselman, W. 1980. *Emma*. New York: Harper and Row.

Koste, V. 1978. *Dramatic Play in Childhood: Rehearsal for Life*. New Orleans: Anchorage Press.

Maclay, E., ed. 1977. *Green Winter: Celebrations of Old Age*. New York: Thomas Y. Crowell Co.

Perschbacher, R. 1984. "An Application of Reminiscence in an Activity Setting: The Tiny Hearts and Aged Hands Program." *The Gerontologist* 24:343-45.

Rice, E. 1959. *The Living Theatre*. New York: Harper and Brothers.

Short, C. 1971. "The Old One and the Wind." In *Understanding Literature*. 1984. New York: Macmillan.

Smith, W. 1973. *Granger's Index to Poetry*. Columbia: New York.

Sohngen, M., and R. Smith. "Images of Old Age in Poetry." 1978. *The Gerontologist* 2:181-86.

Thompson, E. 1979. *On Golden Pond*. New York: Dodd, Mead.

Wertheim, A. 1979. *Radio Comedy*. New York: Oxford University Press.

"Writing the Living Newspaper." 1937. National Service Bureau of Federal Theatre Project of Works Progress Administration.

Wilson, C. 1980. *A Treasure Hunt*. Washington, D.C.: U.S. Department of Health, Education, and Welfare, National Institutes of Health, National Institutes of Aging.

6

Integrated Intergenerational Movement, Dance, and Music

Music and movement have often been referred to as the universal language - the sixth sense, the unspoken language able to move people to tears, to giddiness, to thoughtful moments, to enlightened visions of creativity, or to sadness. "The earliest record of dance comes from the pre-Christian era. The Chaldeans used dance for educational purposes and are credited with the beginning of astronomy, which they taught by means of great symbolic ballets" (T. Marx 1983). For the self-conscious adolescent, movement offers an avenue through which an energized body may move and express important thoughts and ideas. For the senior adult, it is a rediscovered joy. Erna Caplow-Lindner, Leah Harpaz, and Sonya Samber (1979) have found that "geriatric sessions help participants to discover pleasure in moving and through that, to find pleasure in living."

The combination of youth and elderly moving together opens yet another avenue of shared communication. As Gay Hendricks and Kathlyn Hendricks so aptly confirm:

> Another reason for using movement in teaching is to bring people more in harmony with themselves and others. Moving together is a superb way of building community. We all know the unpleasant effects of the lack of a sense of community, whether in a classroom or in the world at large. There is something about dancing and moving with one's fellows that can dissolve the stiffness and alienation that sometimes occurs between humans. In a classroom, teacher and students moving together can build the kind of rapport that is at the heart of meaningful education. (1983, p. 3)

Perhaps one of the most exemplary demonstrations of successful intergenerational movement can be found through the Dance Exchange founded in 1976 in Washington, D.C., by Liz Lerman. In describing past performances of the group, Lerman and C. Reeverts (1981) reported senior citizens, young children, and a young adult as the intergenerational mix of nonprofessionals who performed with the regular company members. A further extension of the Dance Exchange is Dancers of the Third Age consisting of members who are "sixty years of age and more" (McCutcheon and Wolf, p. 136). An excellent source for incorporating dance in any program is Lerman's text, *Teaching Dance to Senior Adults* (1984).

Yet another exemplary program of successful intergenerational dance is that of the Mt. View Elementary School (see Chapter 2). J. Metal-Corbin, D. Corbin, and G. Barker (1986) again stress the values in shared movement experiences between the generations.

Permission to move in a nonmoving society is perhaps the most difficult task in preparing people for dance; thus, the choice of music becomes a prime consideration. Adolescents naturally respond to rock 'n' roll. Some forty- year olds who are still "in-tune" will respond to some of the same music, the Beatles, for example. Their bodies may remember what the adolescent is presently discovering. Somewhere in the middle of these musical life experiences, the adolescent and the middle-aged meet in a shared adventure of joyful movement.

This shared adventure with the elderly may take on a new focus as the adolescent or child is introduced to big band sounds, ballads, country, classical, and religious music. The rhythms are different from the familiar beats of rock music. Thus, as the body movements change, responses to each other are altered, as the communication process takes on a different dimension. New messages are discovered together in a world of music unfamiliar to the young person and movement unfamiliar to the elderly. Most nursing homes have physical therapists and/or exercise programs that involve residents in movement. But, even as middle-aged adults, people are not generally accustomed to recreational movement or movement expression throughout a lifetime. The surge of aerobics has probably done much to promote an interest in moving to music. Yet, aerobics programs did not begin to take full charge until most of the elderly residents were already living in a reassigned residence. Therefore, movement to music or sounds may still be a new experience for many. Often times, people are hesitant to move to music with which they are unfamiliar; yet, once they begin to move, the rhythms become natural and the movement "feels good." The experience is comparable to sitting and listening to a song when all of a sudden a foot begins tapping or fingers begin to snap. Movement to music is a natural act, but one which is usually limited to an evening out, a special occasion, or a weekly aerobics or exercise class. Movement for enjoyment or communication is a rarity, yet one in which the benefits are spiritual, physical, and emotional. It is unfortunate that the only population usually involved in such experiences is performance artists who are either in training or maintaining conditioning for maximum performance capabilities.

For the actor/artist the body becomes the tool through which he or she communicates and creates. For the individual the body becomes a nonverbal form of communication not only to others but to oneself as well. It follows suit, then, that the most natural way to begin without inhibiting the body, is to get to know oneself through a series of exercises and a variety of movement experiences.

DANCE AND MOVEMENT EXERCISES

Because we are working with special populations in nursing homes, it is advisable first to consult with the physical therapist, nursing staff, or physicians regarding the individual needs and capabilities of residents before beginning dance and movement experiences.

Body/Self Shared Exercises

1. Hold your hands out in front of you and study them. Try to describe them. Are the fingers long, short, rounded, slender, wide?
2. Stretch your arms out in front of you. Compare the length of your arms with your partner's.
3. In a sitting position compare heights.
4. In a sitting position stretch arms above head and compare.
5. In a sitting position stretch your legs out in front of you and compare leg lengths.
6. Repeat all the preceding steps to the sound of music or to beats.
   a. hands out in front with fingers spread, go back to neutral position, hands back at waist
   b. stretch arms above head, return to neutral position
   c. outstretch arms, return to neutral position
   d. outstretch legs, return to neutral position

Variations in Music

1. Repeat preceding exercises, but change music several times.

2. After each music change, have participants talk about the different ways in which people in the group moved.

Music That Suggests Themes

1. Select music that suggests themes, such as "Appalachian Spring" by Aaron Copland.

2. Create a "movement scene" using improvisational theatre techniques. The scene should be based upon whatever theme the music implies and should be nonverbal.

Scarfs as a Movement Extension

1. Again, select music with a theme.

2. Use scarfs or lightweight strips of fabric to move to the music.

Shadow Dancing

1. Use an overhead projector and screen to create silhouettes.

2. Add poetry readings to the silhouette shadows.

Expressive Movement

Supplies include notecards, markers, selections of music from various genres.

1. Have participants write words that designate feelings on the notecards. Words such as sad, happy, confused, surprised, and angry provide recognizable motivators, as most people have experienced these emotions.

2. Have participants divide into groups. Group A
arranges Group B in a still sculpture that represents the
word on the notecard.

3. Have participants slowly bring the "still sculpture" to
life.

4. Gradually add music to the piece, and have
participants continue to add movements as they listen
and respond to the music and to each other.

5. Variation: have watching group try to guess the word
the performing group has drawn.

Working Symphony

1. Participants sit in a circle. One participant begins
movement of arm, finger, leg, head, or shoulders.
Person sitting next to leader adds another movement;
the next person adds another movement until the entire
circle of participants are moving.

2. Variation: Participants may add sounds with the
movement.

The advantage to vocal exercise is that those who may have a minimal
capacity for movement but have the use of the voice may be able to contribute
sound to the ensemble, thus continuing involvement with the group. The same
opportunity may hold true for those who have lost use of the voice but still
have movement capabilities. The opportunity for everyone to make a
contribution is vital to the success of the ensemble effect and experience. It is
also an important part of positive self-image (keeping in mind that those who
have lost the use of parts of the body may be frustrated or feel a sense of
inadequacy). Being able to contribute to a group may focus the energy and
mind on the positive rather than on the loss or a negative physical image.
Accentuate the positive!

The advantage to working with residents in nursing homes is the
ability to focus upon specific areas of the body rather than a large picture of
the whole body. Moving the fingers or opening and closing a hand may
become an entire choreographed piece. Children and youth are thus afforded

the opportunity to focus upon specific areas of the body and develop a sense of specificity.   Concentrating on the hand also helps to remove the self-consciousness of the adolescent who is already too painfully aware of his or her changing body.

LABAN TECHNIQUE

Several different theories of study should also be mentioned here, as they may lend further insight into the process of movement and dance. One of the forerunners in movement study was Rudolf Laban, who "sought expression of his art and philosophy amongst ordinary people, and all over Europe centres were established in his name for the craftsmen who came to seek advice on their own working problems and on the strain and stresses involved in their various occupations" (R. Laban and F. C. Lawrence 1974, p. xiii).   Laban developed a system of movement notation known in America as Labanotation. Furthermore, "through his study of mind-body relationships and the psychological effects of certain movement patterns, he was able to achieve improvements in many emotionally disturbed people as well as in those with physical limitations" (p.xiv).   Laban stressed the individual rhythms of people, comparing a "strong, quick and direct" with a "sensitive fine touch, sustained consideration and a flexible approach to decisions and actions" (p.2).

Based on Laban's observations, it might be helpful first to determine the usual methods of movement for each of the participants involved in the class. Although the distinction between strong, quick movements and slow, deliberate ones may be a bit of an over-generalization, it is a good beginning point for students and residents. A two-category checklist of how students and residents approach everyday activities may be an excellent avenue for self-study. A further comparison of the styles of movement partners from the school and from the nursing home would also be helpful in learning to become observant about movements of others.   Perhaps in the summation, understanding the movement patterns of others would enhance communication and shared understanding.   The students and residents may further study movement by considering the rhythmic patterns of characters they develop and portray.

Daily Observation Sheet
Name: Age:
Activity:
Getting out of bed
Time:
5:00 a.m.
Movement Description:
Stretch, slow, lift head slowly, stretch. Respond to music on the clock-radio.

(See Appendix B for worksheet.)

Students and residents may want to brainstorm together to decide upon the various categories to be included in the daily observation sheet. The act of brainstorming and thinking about various categories is, in a sense, a training tool for becoming sensitized to movement observation. Laban and Lawrence also assert that "rhythm speaks to us independently of the task to which it is applied" (p.5).

The act of movement observation should come after the initial experiences with movement exercises in order to motivate interest and further awareness of the body as a rhythmic communicator. Participants, having experienced positive connections with movement, will be more apt to want to further their investigations.

The group may want to expand their study of Laban's methods, including his observations of time, weight, and space. It is possible that these investigations will correspond with lessons in biology and/or mathematics, depending upon the level of the group. Certainly Laban's exercises lend themselves to thoughtful movement and may even lead to creative dance or scene interpretation. For example:

(c)stretching-wringing. Exercise: stretch elastic or cloth
by hand. (p.37)

(a)patting-dabbing. Exercise: pat dough with hand, or
level index cards by hand. (p.37)

Laban's insights into the psychological effects of effort/movement control have a bearing on the understanding of everyday movement. "People moving with easy effort seem to be freer than those moving with obviously stressed effort. The latter seem to struggle against something" (p.62). Laban attributes some of this resistance to the time factor. Youth and residents might then also consider time elements involved in movement.

Another main characteristic that Laban investigated was that of the "presence or lack of bodily force. It is the degree of energy spent in overcoming one's own body weight, or that of an object, which expresses itself in the effort attitude towards the weight factor" (p.63). Laban goes on to discuss elements of movement through space:

> Easy movers might be observed to use a great deal of flexibility and twists in their efforts. That means, they apparently swim, circulate and twist most thoroughly through any possible region of space. Enjoying the space surrounding them makes them happy dwellers of a kingdom of which they know every corner. (pp. 63-4)

Perhaps this last quote is of the greatest importance to the movement/dance participant. When there is an enjoyment of movement, a freedom of physical flow, then the experience becomes one of the highest forms of enjoyment.

> People who indulge in flow find pleasure in the unrestricted freedom of fluency, without necessarily giving much attention to the various shades of the time, the weight and the space development of the movement. Movements with free flow cannot be easily interrupted or suddenly stopped; it takes time until the moving person gains the necessary control over the flow in order to stop. Those persons who tend to bind their flow will be able to stop their movements at any instant. (p. 65)

ALEXANDER TECHNIQUE

Yet another avenue of study is that of the Alexander Principle.

> The Principle proposes a different way of living and of seeing one's life, not different in the sense of making its users into oddities, but different in that its users can learn to adopt other criteria for themselves and for the people they live with. Its users (over the thirty years I have observed it) seem to be able to adapt more

> successfully than most people in their social, artistic, and
> biological spheres. And, most important of all, they
> appear to live longer and more healthily. (Barlow 1973,
> p.3)

Alexander technique places a special emphasis upon the use of the body both in motion and in stillness. Furthermore, Alexander stresses that use affects a person's modes of functioning. Although it is advisable to have a trained Alexander teacher administer lessons to the group, this practice may not be financially feasible. A second approach might be to raise money to provide opportunities for a teacher or teachers to train in this method. The benefits of this type of program for youngsters and the elderly are immeasurable, as there is a renewed sensitivity not only to the participation through movement in classes but in everyday activities as well. With its special attention to comfortable spinal alignment, positioning, and awareness of the various internal and external parts of the body, the participant begins to become aware of healthy postures of physical success, rather than self-consciousness, as in the case of the adolescent, or depression or apathy as experienced by many of the elderly.

The suggestion has been made that children could become more interested in learning through the proper understanding of "end-gaining" as promoted by Alexander technique. John Dewey, American pioneer in education, saw great value in the understanding of inhibiting immediate reaction to a stimulus, thus increasing the possibility of the involvement of quality experience in processing, rather than jumping to an end-gain. The impact of this philosophy not only may be physical but also may be of greater importance as students think through answers and consider various avenues of questioning, reasoning, and investigation, before responding. The focus then becomes one of modeling and providing opportunities for youth to become great thinkers rather than quick reactors. This is not to say that immediate responses to stimuli are unimportant. The speed at which a person may learn a quality response may increase with practice and the correct approach. It is important to consider one of the concepts of aging, entailing the speed at which some elderly respond to stimulus. Up until a few years ago, this lengthened response time was considered a "sign of aging," then went on to become a "myth of aging," until it was finally studied, understood, and reinterpreted by gerontologists and social scientists as reflecting the increased time spent on pondering and evaluation before response. Comparative study between Alexander teachers and gerontologists might lead to yet undiscovered areas of stimulus/response.

Thus, it is important to not only study dance, but the physical state-of-being for each participant. The concept of wellness as a total involvement including both the mind and the body has become increasingly popular among health care providers, diagnosticians, athletes, and those involved with the overall health of human beings. In working with a "holistic" approach to theatre, dance, music, and movement experiences, then, it seems natural to combine all four areas for a total involvement. The first step, however, would be the investigation of the self and then the partner.

SELF-INVESTIGATION

Self-study may be the most difficult exercise of all, as individuals are hesitant to examine themselves in the mirror. However, constant coaching by the teacher to "Study; don't judge!" will help individuals to rid themselves of self-criticism and become self-social scientists. For a change the elderly and the young will have the opportunity to study themselves and come to conclusions regarding their development and movement.

Mirror - Shared Observation

1. Look at your face in the mirror. Does one ear seem to be closer to your shoulder? Which one?

2. Look at the lines on your face. Try to identify the "life experience" that might have earned this line for you. Perhaps you will want to tell the story behind certain lines.

3. Allow "youth-partners" to smile, frown, look puzzled, angry, and hurt. Try to determine where they might develop future face lines.

4. Study the shape of the shoulders. Are your higher than your partner's? Are they rounded? Are they straight across?

5. Study the torso. Is it long? short? What are the lines? Is it concave? Straight up and down?

6. Study the legs. How long are they? Which way do the feet point?

7. Study the length of the arms in relation to the rest of the body. How far down do they hang?

Stimulus-Response

1. Call out various emotions and try to use emotional-physical recall to react physically to each of the stimulus words: tired, confused, happy, sad, fearful, bored. Notice the positions of each of the various external limbs and make note of them. Also include facial expressions.

Musical Stimulus-Response

1. Repeat the exercises above but add various types of music and observe the physical reaction to each type of music.

2. Add finger movements; hand movements; arm movements; head and neck movements; leg movements to the music. Listen to the music first and wait for a physical response.

3. One partner begins a movement to music with the fingers; another partner adds to the movement using another part of the body. This may continue until all are involved in the dance piece.

A word should be said here about the advantages of unplanned or improvisational movement. The body is accustomed, from the fluidity of the womb, to movement - unplanned, natural, uninhibited movement. Movement becomes inhibited only as we pass and are guided by the able hands of a surgeon through the birth canal. It makes sense, then, that we should listen to music and then respond to it through natural movements. In discussing kinesthetic reactions, James Penrod says we possess "three senses through which we are aware of our movements and body. They are the kinesthetic sense, the static sense, and the visceral sense"(1974, pp. 2-3). He equates the kinesthetic sense with control of body positions and movement, while the static sense "gives you information about the position of your body in space, the direction of your movement in space, and the changes in speed of a movement" (p. 3). The visceral sense is connected with functions of the internal organs.

Penrod talks about "experiencing movement dynamically." Having studied his text, one begins to notice the similarities between his philosophy of movement and that of Laban and the Alexander technique. Penrod reviews such terms as "pushing and pulling; resisting and yielding; percussive and sustained action; vibratory (shaking) and slash actions; sliding and gliding; swinging and swaying" (p. 13), all of which are mentioned both by Laban in his notations and Alexander in his "end-gaining" and "inhibiting" (pp. 170-71). It is therefore important that specialists, amateurs, and dancer-musicians look carefully at all three areas before engaging upon choreographed pieces.

It is important for individuals to feel good about their bodies in order to feel good about their bodies in relation to others and to movement with and for others. It is after this initial reorientation to the body/movement/soul that the appropriate time for formalized choreography and dance pieces may be introduced or reintroduced. It is also at this time that the group and individuals will experience a new vitality and an awareness of this phenomenon in life called movement, regardless of the rhythm, beat, mood, or message of the music. The participants will now be more open to understanding various movments and each other, as they move through not only the dance/music class, but life itself.

REFERENCES

Barlow, W. 1973. *The Alexander Technique*. New York: Alfred A. Knopf.

Caplow-Lindner. 1979. *Therapeutic Dance Movement: Expressive Activities for Older Adults*. New York: Human Sciences Press.

Hendricks, G., and K. Hendricks. 1983. *The Moving Center*. Englewood Cliffs, NJ: Prentice Hall.

Laban, R., and Lawrence, F.C. 1974. *Effort: Economy In Body Movement*. Boston: Plays, Inc.

Lerman, L. 1984. *Teaching Dance to Senior Adults*. Springfield, IL: Charles D. Thomas Publishers.

Lerman, L., and C. Reeverts. 1981. "The Dance Exchange" *Design for Arts in Education* 83:11-20.

Marx, T. 1983. *Tap Dance: A Beginner's Guide*. Englewood Cliffs, NJ: Prentice Hall.

Metal-Corbin, J. D., D. Corbin, and G. Barker. 1986. "Age Doesn't Matter: Weaving Dance into a Fifth Grade Curriculum." Paper presented at the National AAHPERD Conference in Cincinnati, Ohio, on April 13.

McCutcheon, P., and C. Wolf. 1985. *The Resource Guide to People, Places, and Programs in the Arts and the Aging*. Washington, D.C.: National Council on the Aging.

Penrod, J. 1974. *Movement for the Performing Artist*. Palo Alto, CA: Mayfield Publishing Company.

Appendix A
Plays

"FANTASY LAND" PLAY OUTLINE
"THE LITTLE OLD BAG LADY" PUPPET PLAY
FILL-IN-THE BLANK MYSTERY PLAY
"SAME BLUE EYES" RADIO PLAY

"FANTASY LAND" PLAY OUTLINE

CHARACTERS: *(Depending upon the costumes the seniors and children have created together, it may be possible to suggest some stock characters.)*

NARRATOR   TOWNSPEOPLE   KING   QUEEN
PRINCE   PRINCESS
THE WISEPERSON   PEOPLE OF THE KING'S COURT   DRAGON

Scene i

Narrator: The townspeople were very sad because the dragon decided to eat all of the storybooks in the land. Without books, the children could not learn and the King could not hear his nightly story.

(Cue: Participants walk around as if they were sad. They may make up dialogue as they walk through the town. The King may groan, and the Queen might wring her hands and moan.)

Narrator: All the King's court and the townspeople tried and tried to cheer up the King, but all he could do was sit and moan!

(Cue: King moans)

(Cue: Participants ad lib as they try to cheer up the King.)

Scene ii

(Cue: Participants sit down after seeing that cheering up the King will be an impossible job.)

(Cue: The Princess jumps up.)

Narrator: The Princess had an idea! She suggested that they call upon the Wiseperson to find a solution.

(Cue: Participants move to a designated area of the room to the Wiseperson.)
Narrator: The townspeople descended upon the Wiseperson, who suggested that they take turns telling the King stories at night and that tonight they begin the first story.

(Cue: The Wiseperson may ad lib the dialogue here.)

(Cue: A designated townsperson holds up a cardboard moon or stars to indicate night time.)

Scene iii

(Cue: One of the townspeople tells a story while the rest act it out. The King becomes very amused, and the townspeople begin to smile again.)

(Cue: The little boy and Wiseperson may actually say the following lines.)

Narrator and/or Little Boy: One of the little boys asked, " I liked the story, but how can we learn if we don't have any books?"

Narrator and/or Wiseperson: The Wiseperson replied, "Tomorrow night, someone will share some knowledge at the Court."

Scene iv

(Cue: A townsperson holds up a cardboard sun and then the moon to indicate the passing of time.)

Narrator: The next evening one of the children told about a history lesson.

(Cue: A townsperson may tell something they learned about history.)

Narrator: The King was very pleased and cheered. The people in the court began to applaud, when all of a sudden one of the elders from the kingdom noticed something glowing in the corner.

(Cue: Participants cheer but then become very quiet.)

(Cue: The participant playing the Prince may say the following line.)

Narrator and/or Prince: The brave Prince approached the light and said, "Halt! Who goes there?"

Narrator: Very slowly and sheepishly, the dragon appeared. At first everyone was frightened but the dragon begged the people to stay and listen to his story.

Dragon: Every night I listen to the King's stories, and every day I hear the children laughing in school. I am an old dragon with no place to go and I love to hear stories and learn. That's why I ate all your books *(Burp!)*. Won't you please let me stay, and I promise never to eat any more of your books!

Narrator: The townspeople thought about the dragon's request and then the Wiseperson came forward.

(Cue: The townspeople should walk around and appear to be thinking.)

Wiseperson: Of course you can stay, but you must first teach us something and tell us a story.

Narrator: And with that the townspeople cheered and gathered around the dragon to hear his story.

(Cue: Participants circle around the Dragon and hold up their arms to take a bow as they announce:
                              THE END!

Note: The instructors/teachers may want to ask a senior or young student to decide before the play upon a topic for the short lesson and a short story or joke to be incorporated into scenes iii and iv.

Participants may also elect to invent character names and a name for the kingdom. The decision for a title may be made either before or after the performance. Sometimes the decision for a title is best left for the end, as discussion concerning the choice usually follows.

"THE LITTLE OLD BAG LADY"

CHARACTERS:

BAG LADY   BOY   GIRL   WIZARD

The Bag Lady appears on stage right. She is very upset and pacing about)

Bag Lady: Oh, dear! Oh, dear. If I don't find my bag I shall never get home.

Boy: (Appears on the opposite side of the stage) Gosh! If I don't find that dollar I lost, Mom's going to be really angry!

(They move to the center of the stage, bumping into each other.)

Both: Ouch!

Boy: I'm sorry. I didn't see you!

Bag Lady: Oh, today's just not my day!

Boy: Mine neither.

Bag Lady: Well, what happened to you?

Boy: My mother gave me a dollar to buy some milk, and I lost it on the way to the store. I'm always losing things!

Bag Lady: Me too.

Boy: Yeah, but I bet your mom doesn't yell at you.

Bag Lady: No, but the Wizard will when he finds out I've lost the bag!

Boy: The what?

Bag Lady: The bag! The bag! It contains all our earthly belongings! Everything we own, and I had to lose it!

Boy: Gosh! All in one bag? Well, what did it look like? Maybe I could help you look for it.

Bag Lady: Well, I guess that would be helpful to have an extra set of eyes. Are you sure you don't mind?

Boy: No, but maybe you could help me look for my dollar.

Bag Lady: It's a deal!

Boy: Well, the first thing to do is to retrace your steps. That's what my mother always says, anyway.

Bag Lady: Really? That's what the Wizard always says, too.

(They both begin to exit stage right as the Girl and the Wizard enter stage left.)

Girl: Are you sure you lost it here?

Wizard: I'm sure! I had the bag in my hand. I put it beside this bush here, and when I turned around it was gone! Oh, how could I have lost the bag! Of all the things to lose!

Girl: But maybe you didn't lose it. Maybe you just misplaced it. That's what my mom says all the time.

Wizard: Oh, you're very nice to help me, but I don't think I'll ever be able to find it again!

Girl: Well, one more time....let's retrace your steps and see if we can find it.

Wizard: Oh, alright. But I don't think this is going to work!

(The Girl and the Wizard walk backward from one side of the stage, while the Boy and the Bag Lady walk backward from the other side of the stage. The four meet in the middle with a BUMP!)

All: OUCH! OUCH! OUCH! OUCH!

(As soon as they recover they recognize each other. The boy and girl are sister and brother, and the Bag Lady recognizes the Wizard as her husband.)

Bag Lady: Oh, I have the most terrible news!

Wizard: No, wait, before you tell your news, let me tell you mine!

Boy: Well, I have bad news, too.

Wizard: It can't be as bad as mine.

Boy: Worse.

Bag Lady: No mine is just awful!

Girl: What is everybody so upset about?

Boy: I lost the dollar mom gave me.

Bag Lady: I lost the bag!

Wizard: You lost the bag?

Bag Lady: (crying) Yes, I lost the bag!

Wizard: I thought I lost the bag.

Girl: You didn't lose your dollar. I found it on the kitchen counter. You left it at home.

Boy: I did?

Girl: I came after you, but you had already left. Then I met up with Mr. Wizard, who lost his bag, and I said I'd help him. Have you seen a bag?

Boy: No. But we've been looking for one.

Bag Lady: Oh, dear, now we won't have a place to live.

Wizard: That bag and everything in it was our home.

Girl: You mean you don't have a home?

Bag Lady and Wizard (Both shaking their heads): No.

Boy: Hey, I've got an idea!

Girl: Me too!

(Boy and Girl go off and whisper to each other. Then they jump up and down with excitement.)

Boy: My sister and I think you should come home and live with us.

Bag Lady: Oh, no, we couldn't do that.

Girl: Oh, please. We have enough room, and our mother is always saying she wished we had some help.

Wizard: Well, maybe we could...just until we found our bag, of course.

Bag Lady: We could stay for a short time while we looked for our bag. Yes. I think we could.

Boy and Girl: Yeah!

(As the four are going off together)

Girl: *(to Bag Lady)* I'll share my room with you.

Boy: *(to Wizard)* I'll let you sleep in the top bunk! Say, what did you say was in that bag anyway?

Wizard: Oh, nothing, really, just a wish...a wish for a home.

FILL-IN-THE-BLANK MYSTERY

The Case of the Missing ————————————————————
(fill in the blank)

Characters:

NARRATOR
CHARACTER #1 (PRIVATE INVESTIGATOR)
CHARACTER #2 (PRIVATE INVESTIGATOR)
CHARACTER #3 (MYSTERY PERSON)

Narrator: It was cold and ——————————————— *(Describe the night.)*

the night of *(Provide a date.)*

————————————————— when the office of private

investigators, *(Provide a name for Character #1.)*

————————————————————————————

and *(Provide a name for Character #2.)*

————————————————————————————

received a very mysterious phone call. It seems that *(Fill in the*

details for the phone call.)

————————————————————————————

————————————————————————————

————————————————————————————

————————————————————————————

————————————————————————————

----------------------------------!!!!!!

Character #1 (Private Investigator): I can't believe this. Why only a minute ago

we--

Character #2 (Private Investigator): I know, I know. But there **must** be a

reason why this would happen. I wonder if....

Character #1: If what? If what?!!!

Character #2: Did you hear that???!! Shhhhh!!!

Character #1: I think it's...I think it's...

Character #2: You're right! It's *(Description of the*

intruder)----------------------------------

Character #1: Wait! I think I've got a plan.

Character #2: What? What's your plan?

Character #1: Okay. Now listen very carefully. Let's *(Fill in an idea for a*

plan.)

Character #2: Okay, and then let's *(Add to Character #1's plan.)*

Character #1: But what if

(They both freeze as Character #3 enters.)

Character #3 (You provide the name.): Fancy meeting you here.

Character #1: Now, wait a second. You told us you were

_____

_____

_____

_____

Character #3: Oh, I did but I

_____

_____

_____

_____

_____

_____–instead!

Character #2: Well, what have you got to say for yourself?

Character #3: Not much.

Character #1: If that's the case then we're all going to have to *(Fill in an idea*

for another plan.)

_____

_____

_____

_____

_____

Narrator: Strange, but true. For the next five years the

_ _

_ -! And

the other turned out to be none other than

_ _

_ _

_ _

THE END

"SAME BLUE EYES"

CHARACTERS:

PRISON GUARD (AROUND FORTY-FIVE YEARS OF AGE. HE IS STERN YET
        SYMPATHETIC.)
INMATE #1 (CATMAN) (ABOUT FORTY, BLACK, INCARCERATED SINCE THE
        AGE OF EIGHTEEN. HE LOVES TO SING AND LAUGH.)
INMATE #2 (ABOUT TWENTY-THREE, PLAYS THE HARMONICA)
PETE SLADEN (ABOUT SIXTY-FIVE, FROM A SMALL SOUTHERN TOWN)
KELLY SLADEN (ABOUT EIGHTEEN YEARS OF AGE, RECENTLY GRANDUATED
        FROM HIGH SCHOOL AND COLLEGE BOUND)

SETTING:

A prison work farm

Scene i - Cell block sixteen
Scene ii - The chapel in the prison

SUGGESTIONS FOR PRODUCTION MUSIC:

Gotta' Serve Somebody by Bob Dylan
Harmonica Music
At end of show, *Simple Twist of Fate* by Bob Dylan, as sung by Joan Baez on
the *Diamonds and Rust* Album

*SFX: SOUND OF CLANGING STEEL GATES OF A PRISON ARE
HEARD; PERHAPS KEYS IN A LOCK AND THE SLAMMING OF
ANOTHER SET OF GATES*

Prison Guard: Mail call!

Inmate #1: Anything from my wife?

Inmate #2: Catman, when was the last time you heard from your wife? You
        ain't even got a wife. You've been locked up so long you gone
        plumb crazy!

Prison Guard: Gramps! You got a letter.

Pete: I got a letter? Must be some kinda' mistake.

Prison Guard: Says right here, "Mr. Peter Sladen." You're the only Peter Sladen locked up here. Here you go, Gramps.

Pete: Well, I'll be. Thanks.

SFX: SOUND OF LETTER BEING OPENED

SFX: INMATE CALLING FROM A CELL FURTHER AWAY

Inmate #1: Hey, Gramps, you got a secret love on the outside you ain't told us about?

SFX: LAUGHTER FROM THE OTHER INMATES

Inmate #2: Yeah, Catman, your wife!

SFX: LAUGHTER AND WHISTLING FROM THE OTHER INMATES

Prison Guard: Alright, you guys, settle down. Let the old man read his mail. Hope it ain't bad news, Gramps.

Pete: No, no. It's from... someone I've never met.

Prison Guard: You advertise for a pen pal or something?

Pete: No, this is a special letter. This is from my grandson, Kelly. My grandson I've never even seen.

Prison Guard: Well, ain't you gonna' read it?

Pete: *(He is in a mixed state of shock, happiness, sadness, and wonderment.)* Yes. Yes, I guess I'd better read it.

Inmate #1: Well, ain't you gonna' tell us what it says?

Pete: It says...he wants to visit me. After all these years, he wants to talk to me. He wants to visit me.

Prison Guard: How old is he?

Pete: Kelly?...He must be...oh, maybe eighteen, maybe twenty....I don't know, I lost track. Kelly...my grandson, Kelly.

Inmate #1: What else does the letter say?

Pete: Not much. Just that his parents don't know that he's comin', but he has something important to talk to me about.

Prison Guard: You know, Gramps, after all these years of knowin' ya' I never knew you had a family, much less a grandson.

Pete: Oh, yeah, I got a fine family. My son's a bigwig manager or something like that with a construction firm. Course I haven't talked to him in maybe twenty years. Maybe thirty. His grandmother, Emily, my ex, wouldn't allow any of the family to contact me. Might say she disowned me....

Inmate #2: Yeah, don't they all. "For better or for worse." But when it's for the worse they don't want nothin' to do with ya'.

Pete: I don't know what I'll have to say to him. His mother and grandmother'd be mighty mad to know he came to see me. Maybe I'd better tell him "no." After all these years I'm better off to the family forgotten.

Prison Guard: Yeah, but Gramps, if the kid wants to see ya', let him see ya'. Can't do that much harm. After all, you're locked up. (*They both laugh.*)

Pete: Yeah, I'm locked up. Other grandfathers take their grandsons fishin'. Take 'em to baseball games. Me? I'm locked up. Nah.... I'm gonna' tell the kid "no." What have I got to offer him? Nothing. Nothing.

Prison Guard: Don't forget, this is a prison farm. We got the fishin' hole down the hill. I bet if you talked to the warden, he might consider givin' you permission to take the kid fishin'. I mean as long as one of us guards was along with you.

Inmate #1: Hey, Gramps, you forget about the baseball game next Saturday? Remember, we're gonna' beat the pants offa' cell block eighteen.

Inmate #2: Yeah, say, we got baseball here. Darn good baseball! Bet your grandkid never seen a bunch a' cons play ball before. Now that's something to see!

Inmate #1: Yeah, we play for blood! *(Laughter from everyone.)*

Pete: *(Laughing.)* Yeah, you're right. We got a good ball club here. A *good* ball club. *(Pause.)* I don't know. I just don't know. If I was a businessman, or a teacher, or a bricklayer, *something*, I'd feel better about seein' him. Anything but a convict...a con.

Prison Guard: An honest convict, Gramps! Remember, you're a model prisoner.

Pete: *(Half-laughing.)* Yeah, a model prisoner. Better 'n' nothin', I suppose. I don't know, I'll have to think about it.

SFX: *A HARMONICA IS HEARD IN THE BACKGROUND. A BLACK MAN BEGINS TO SING A PRISON SONG. SOFTLY.*

Pete: I'll have to give it some thought.

SFX: *HARMONICA AND SINGING BECOME MORE DISTINCT AS OTHER INMATES JOIN IN. MUSIC BECOMES LOUDER AND THEN FADES OUT.*

SFX: *THE CLANGING OF HEAVY GATES AND THE SOUND OF KEYS. IT IS SCENE II AND VISITING DAY.*

Prison Guard: Alright, Gramps. This is your big day. Your visitor's here.

Pete: Alright, I'm almost ready.

Inmate #1: He's been in his cell primpin' for the last two hours. You'd think he had a hot date or somethin'!

Pete: I even put my teeth in!

Inmate #1: Whoa!!!

Inmate #2: Even put his teeth in!!! *(Laughter from other inmates and Guard.)*

Prison Guard: Alright, you two, knock it off! This is Gramp's special day. He's nervous enough without the two of you razzin' him. Come on, old man, hurry it up in there. You're losin' precious time with your grandson!

SFX: WE HEAR THE GUARD'S KEYS UNLOCK PETE'S CELL. THE PRISON GUARD WHISTLES AS HE SEES PETE.

Prison Guard: Whew! Just look at you all slicked up!

Pete: Well, like you said, this is a special day. I want to make a good impression on my grandson.

Inmates #1 & #2: (Whistling.) Whew, look at Gramps!

Inmate #1: Hey, Gramps, you look twenty years younger! Smile for us....Let us see your teeth! I never seen you with your teeth in before!

Pete: How's this?

(Inmates and Guard laugh and clap.)

Inmate #1: Hey, Gramps....

Pete: Yeah, Catman?

Inmate #1: (For the first time he is sincere.) I hope everything goes alright for you.

Inmate #2: Yeah, tell that grandson of yours that we said he's got the best darn grandfather anybody could ask for.

Pete: Thanks.

Prison Guard: Okay, Pete, we'd better get going.

SFX: SOUNDS OF FOOTSTEPS AS THEY WALK DOWN THE HALL. PERHAPS THE SOUND OF ONE OR TWO GATES OPENING AND CLOSING.

Prison Guard: Okay, Gramps. He's inside the chapel there. Warden said to give you fifteen minutes, then your time's up. Sorry it's such a short time, but regulations, you know.

Pete: Oh, sure, that's okay. *(Pause.)* Didn't think I'd be this nervous. All these years I never had a visitor. *(Hesitating.)* Well..., I guess I'd better go in.

SFX: THE SOUND OF A DOOR SLOWLY OPENING AND CLOSING.

Pete: *(Pausing for a moment.)* Hi. My name's Pete Sladen. I guess you must be Kelly.

Kelly: Yessir. That's me.

SFX: THE SOUND OF FOOTSTEPS AS THEY WALK TOWARD EACH OTHER

Pete: Well, it's nice to meet you after all these years, Kelly.

Kelly: Thank you, sir. *(There is an awkward silence and Pete clears his throat.)*

Pete: Say, let's sit down over here by the window. I like to see out the windows as much as possible here.

(He makes a feeble attempt at a joke, and Kelly makes a feeble attempt to laugh.)

SFX: THE SOUND OF THE TWO PULLING OUT CHAIRS FROM A TABLE AND SITTING.

Pete: Looks like a pretty nice day out.

Kelly: Yessir. It's a nice day outside. Not too hot, least for the end of June.

Pete: Yessir, we been lucky with the weather this year. It can get pretty hot inside these walls in the summer. But this year we been pretty lucky.

Kelly: Yessir, weather's been good, for this time a year and all....

(Kelly is obviously nervous, and Pete is having a difficult time talking.)

Pete: Ever been inside a prison before, son?

Kelly: No, sir. This is my first time. *(Kelly is obviously relieved to talk about this experience, and some of the ice is broken.)* I didn't know I'd have to be searched and all. I mean, I guess I knew they'd have to check me to make sure I wasn't bringin' anthing in, but I've never been searched before. It was kinda' scarey.

Pete: Yeah, I imagine so. Sorry you had to go through that, son. *(Pause.)* Were the guards nice to you? They didn't cause you any problems or nothin' did they?

Kelly: Oh, no, sir, they were very nice. I guess I must have looked pretty scared and they took pity on me. *(He laughs.)*

Pete: (Laughing as well) Yeah, you should o' seen me the first day I came to prison. I bet I was more scared than you were. *(They both laugh.)* Course, I came in under different circumstances. I had reason to be scared.

Kelly: Yessir.

Pete: Now this is home and I ain't scared anymore. It's not a bad place. Heck, I get free rent and board and clothes. Can't beat that, now, can you, son?

Kelly: No, sir. I wish I could get free room and board. Mom and Dad make me pay them a little each week. I'm tryin' to save for college at the same time. It's tough.

Pete: Oh, goin' to college are ya'?

Kelly: Yessir! *(He's proud to tell about this.)* I got a partial scholarship to the state university.

Pete: Oh, a scholarship, huh? What kind of a scholarship? *(Pete can't help but show that he is becoming a proud grandfather very quickly.)*

Kelly: In math, sir. I plan to go into computers.

Pete: (Whistles.) In math. *(Laughs.)* My grandson, the math wiz! Well, your father was always good in math, so I hear. I expect you picked that up from him.

Kelly: I suppose so. *(There is an awkward silence.)*

Pete: Folks know your here, Kelly?

Kelly: No, sir. They...they wouldn't understand.

Pete: Yeah, I know. Your grandmother never forgave me, did she? Never could forgive me after all these years. Oh, I tried. For a while I wrote to her every week. Just like steady clockwork, but she never wrote back. But I heard all about your father and then you, of course. You still get news on the inside here, ya' know. Somebody knows somebody else, or somebody's cousin is locked up here. *(Pause.)* Oh, I knew all about the day you was born! Even sent a special letter to your dad. But of course he never answered back. 'Spect your grandmother kinda' turned him against me.

Kelly: I'm sorry, sir, I really am. *(Short pause.)* I found your letters to grandmama and I read them all. She doesn't know I read them. She asked me to help clean out her attic one day, and I just came across them. I knew they were private and everything, but I just couldn't help myself. They seemed to be a part of my past that nobody would ever tell me about...and, well, I felt I had a right to know.

Pete: Yes, you did have a right to know. *(Pause.)* Your grandmother kept all my letters, did she? *(Pete can't hide his pleasure.)*

Kelly: Oh, yessir. It looked like she kept every single one of them. They were all bundled together nice and neat with yellow and blue and red ribbons, all arranged and color-coded by the years.

Pete: Well, that would be about right. I gave up after three years of writin' and never hearin' anything.

Kelly: I read all about the accident, sir.

Pete: Ah, well. That was a long time ago. The accident. A long, long time ago.

Kelly: Well, sir, I hope you don't mind, and you can say 'no' to this if you want to, but one of the reasons I wanted to come and see you was to ask about...about....

Pete: You want to know about the accident don't you?

Kelly: *(Quietly)* Yessir.

Pete: Well, I supppose I at least owe you that much. You got just as much right to know why your old granpa's been locked up all these years....I don't even know where to begin....You'll have to excuse me...after all these years...and it's hard to talk with these blasted teeth in my mouth. I usually don't wear them. *(They both laugh.)* Well, let's see. Your grandma and I were friends in school. Oh, she was a looker, your grandma. Most popular girl at Rapids School.

Kelly: Grandmama was a looker, huh? *(Both laugh.)*

Pete: Oh, yeah. I think everybody in the whole school was in love with your grandma. Especially me! I tried everything I could to get her attention. I went out for sports....I was pretty good, too. But she was dating Elmer Harley....

Kelly: Of the "Harley Sporting Goods" stores?

Pete: Yeah, that's the one. That family always had money. And ole Elmer could always impress the girls with his money. Didn't have much of a brain and even less manners, but he had money. *(Pause.)* Well, it was the spring of our last year in school, and I guess your grandmother had been dating Elmer pretty heavily for going on two years. Then all of a sudden they broke up. And you never wanna' see a more broken heart than your grandmother had. Why, she walked around the school like she'd been hit by a truck or somethin'. Then one day, which was actually the luckiest day of my life, I found her cryin' her eyes out, enough tears comin' outta' her big blue eyes to fill the Atlantic....I'll never forget it. Her sittin' under that big Elm tree in Liberty Park, just cryin'. You know that park, son? Is it still there?

Kelly: Oh, yessir. I go there myself sometimes.

Pete: Well, I sat down beside her, and she seemed ashamed to be caught like that. I don't know where I got the nerve to put my arms around her, but something inside my heart told me it would be okay, so I did. We didn't talk for a long time. I just sat there with my arms around her, holdin' her, and she just kept cryin'. Finally she was able to talk and I guess she was just so glad to have somebody to talk to and was so upset that she just let it all spill out. *(Slight pause.)* Now, you're probably gonna' find this hard to believe and I don't even know if I should be tellin' you alla' this....

Kelly: You can tell me, sir.

Pete: Well, that rascal of a goat, Elmer Harley, had gottn your grandmother pregnant and then just walked out on her. Your grandmother would kill me if she knew I told you alla' this....

Kelly: You mean my...my....

Pete: That's right, son. Your dad's real father was Elmer Harley.

Kelly: No wonder grandmama never wants to talk about the past.

Pete: Well, son, I'm sorry, but it's the truth. When I found out what Elmer had done, I was fightin' mad, but the most important thing to me was to sweep your grandmother up in my arms and marry her just as fast as I could....Heck, I'd been in love with her since grade school...*(laughs)*...since I first chased her around the playground with a frog and threatened to give her warts. I was so in love with that little woman I couldn't see straight. I don't think your grandmother had any choice but to say "yes." I mean there she was pregnant and all...at a time when a girl who wasn't married had no business at all even thinkin' about bein' pregnant...so she accepted and we were married the week after we graduated. I don't know if she loved me at first, but I think she kinda' grew to love me on account of how I sorta' rescued her. And oh, I loved her...I'd been waitin' for her all my life...and here I finally had her and a little baby to boot.

Kelly: The baby was my father.

Pete: The baby was your father.

Kelly: He never told me any of this.

Pete: I expect your father might not even know alla' this. Your grandmother's a mighty proud woman, ya' know.

Kelly: Yeah, I know.

Pete: Well, we was a pretty happy couple for awhile there. But things got to be awful hard with the Depression on and all. I guess your father was about five or so, and I couldn't find any work nowheres. I decided maybe I cvould go into some sorta' fishin' business up by the lake and that way I'd at least have fish for my family to eat...if nothin' else. So, one day, I was mindin' my own business and had gone to Harley's Sports Store to see how much it might cost to get me started with some equipment....That was the worst day of my life.

Kelly: That was the day of the accident.

Pete: That was the day of the accident. These two strange-lookin' men came into the store and pulled a gun on the woman behind the counter, who was Elmer's new wife. They wanted all the money from the register. Elmer Harley came out from the back to see what all the commotion was about, and they shot him. Everything happened so fast that I can't even remember some of the details, but I tried to stop one of them, the one with the gun, when the gun went off and hit Elmer again and then his wife square in the chest. The two men didn't take any money, they just run out the back of the store. Then all of a sudden there were people from all over the place, runnin' and screamin'. The two men had run off, and somehow I was left holdin' the gun lookin' down at Elmer's body. Course you know how that musta' looked to people. *(Pete lets out a long sigh and pauses.)* Everybody knew that Elmer and I had it out for each other...and to Elmer's new wife she thought I had shot Elmer and then tried to shoot her, that I was part of the other two men. *(Pause.)* Well, Mrs. Harley just had a bullet graze her, something like a miracle, 'cause she shoulda' been dead, but Elmer wasn't so lucky, he died about a week later. He lived long enough to testify against me and then along with his wife's story....

Kelly: But couldn't you explain this to someone?

Pete: Well, that family had a lot of money, and they always had it out for me, probably 'cause they thought I'd tell the truth about the baby, and they didn't want the family name dirtied...but they were wrong. I never woulda' told anybody, though I think everybody kinda' suspected anyways. So, I got locked up. And your grandmother, well, some friends took her and your father in. I think it broke her heart. She was awful young and awful scared, and I guess she thought she had to do something right, after the baby and all, so she just put me outta' her life.

Kelly: What happened to the two guys?

Pete: They never caught them. If they coulda' caught 'em I mighta' been cleared up, but, heck, I didn't have enough money to feed my family, much less hire some fancy lawyer.

Kelly: So you've been in prison all these years, and you were really innocent? Didn't you ever come up for parole?

Pete: Oh, after awhile I did. But I was no model prisoner then. I was so mad at the world that I got into more trouble inside the walls then I ever was in outside the prison. Here I was with a wife and a little boy I loved so much, just taken away from me...just ripped away...without even havin' a chance to defend myself...no chance at all against the Harley family. So I was denied parole over and over. They thought I was a real hardened criminal, and as long as the Harley family was around, they made certain I stayed put.

SFX: KNOCK AT THE DOOR

Prison Guard: Gramps, your time is up, sorry.

Pete: Okay, thanks.

Kelly: Well, I guess this means I gotta' go, huh?

Pete: Yes, son, they're pretty strict about the rules around here.

Kelly: He called you, "Gramps."

Pete: *(Laughing.)* Yeah, I'm "Gramps" to all the younger ones around here. Guess I'm the closest thing to a grandpa they got.

Kelly: Well, since you're the closest thing I got to a grandfather would it be okay if I called you "Gramps?"

Pete: *(Laughing)* Yeah, that'd be fine, son. Be a lot better than "sir." I don't know who you're talking to when you say "Sir." *(They both laugh.)*

Kelly: Maybe I could come back next weekend. There's a lot I'd like to you talk about.

Pete: Well, that'd be fine with me. Lord knows I could use some company from the outside. Especially if it's family.

Kelly: I'd like that too.

Pete: Course, I don't want to go causin' any more family problems. I caused your grandmother enough problems already. I don't know. Maybe it's not such a good idea....

Kelly: Look, I'm eighteen years old. I'm an adult. I want to see you. The rest of the family can do and feel whatever they want to....Me, I want to see you, we have a lot to talk about.

Pete: You got the same determination as your grandma, son. Same blue eyes...same sparkle.

Kelly: Next weekend, then?

Pete: *(After some hesitation.)* Alright. Next weekend it'll be. Oh, hey, there's a baseball game here next weekend. Some of the families are comin'. You ever seen a bunch of cons play ball, son?

Kelly: No, sir!!

Pete: Well, wait until you see our ball club play! It's our cell block against block eighteen and you'll see some real serious playin'! Yessirreee!!

Prison Guard: Okay, time's up! Last call! Sorry, Gramps, but it's regulations.

Kelly I'll be back next weekend for the ball game...GRAMPS! *(They both laugh.)*

Pete: Alright, yessir!!!

Prison Guard: Let's go, Gramps.

Pete: Okay. Next weekend, son. See You then!

*SFX:THE SOUND OF THE PRISON GUARD AND PETE WALKING
       DOWN THE CORRIDOR. PETE SUDDENLY REMEMBERS
       SOMETHING AND CALLS BACK TO HIS GRANDSON.*

Pete: Oh, hey, we got a fishin' hole here, too. I could take you fishin' on
          Saturday. You like fishin', boy?

Kelly: *(Calls back.)* I love fishin', Gramps!

Pete: Alright! Alright! I'll take my grandson fishin', then. My grandson the
          math wiz!

*SFX: WE HEAR THE FIRST SET OF IRON GATES CLOSE BEHIND
        THEM AND THE SOUND OF FOOTSTEPS CONTINUES.
        PETE IS QUIETLY CRYING.*

Pete: *(To the Prison Guard)* I got me one heck of a grandson. He's got a
          math scholarship...gonna' be a computer wiz....

Prison Guard: He's a fine lookin' boy, Gramps. Fine lookin' boy.

Pete: That's my grandson...my grandson...Kelly Sladen...my grandson.

*SFX: HE IS STILL CRYING AS WE HEAR THE LAST OF THE IRON
        GATES SLAM SHUT.*

*MUSIC: "SIMPLE TWIST OF FATE," BY BOB DYLAN AS SUNG BY JOAN
        BAEZ ON THE "DIAMONDS AND RUST" ALBUM.*

Appendix B
Charts/Worksheets

LIVING NEWSPAPER RESEARCH FORM
LIVING NEWSPAPER CRITIQUE
LIVING NEWSPAPER PROGRESSION
LIVING NEWSPAPER FORM—HEROES OF THE PAST,
PRESENT, AND FUTURE
INTERGENERATIONAL MAJOR/MINOR CHARACTER
RELATIONSHIPS
RITES OF PASSAGE
DREAMS
CHANGE
HEROISM/COWARDICE
TRIALS AND TRIBULATIONS
VISIONS
DAILY OBSERVATION SHEET

Living Newspaper Research Form

Name: Age: Date:

1. Editor's Name	Age

2. Head Dramatist	Age

3. Lawyer's Name	Age

4. Main Topic

5. Area of Assigned Research

6. List sources you have found in the library:

Title	Author

Living Newspaper Research Form (continued)

7. Read at least one page of research for each source and give a summary below:

Source:
Source:
Source:

8. Interview at least two people (one your own age and one senior citizen) concerning their opinion of or knowledge about the topic.

Name of interviewee #1
Age
Information

Living Newspaper Research Form (continued)

Name of Interviewee #2

Age

Information

9. Write a proposed scene treatment regarding your collected research:

Scene Treatment

LIVING NEWSPAPER CRITIQUE

Title:

Participants:

1. Written work

POINTS---------

2. Rehearsal/Classwork

POINTS---------

3. Script work

POINTS --------

4. Presentation

POINTS---------   TOTAL POINTS----------

FINAL GRADE--------

LIVING NEWSPAPER PROGRESSION

Theme
Managing Producer/ Federal Theatre Project District Director/ Federal Theatre Project National Director

Round-table Discussion
Board of Editors/ Managing Editor

Breaks Down Subject Into Scenes Indicates Treatment
Head Dramatist

Coordinates and Edits Research
City Editor
Research Staff

Writes and Checks Scripts
Managing Editor/ Head Dramatist/ Project Lawyer

Produces and Performs Scripts
Production Manager Director/ Designers/ Actors

LIVING NEWSPAPER
HEROES OF THE PAST, PRESENT, AND FUTURE

	Past	Present	Future
Name			
Birthplace			
Educational background			
Family background Sources of information/ research			
Short scene description			

INTERGENERATIONAL MAJOR/MINOR CHARACTER RELATIONSHIPS

Title:

Author:

Publication Information:

MAJOR CHARACTERS

1. Name:	Age:
2. Name:	Age:

MINOR CHARACTERS

3. Name:	Age:
4. Name:	Age:
5. Name:	Age:

KEY SENTENCES, PHRASES, OR ACTIONS WHICH INDICATE RELATIONSHIPS

1.
2.
3.
4.
5.

RITES OF PASSAGE

Name: Age:

I knew I had come of age and was given more responsiblity when:

Age	Year	Description of Incident

My mother/father knew he/she had come of age and was given more responsibility when:

Age	Year	Description of Incident

My grandfather/grandmother knew he/she had come of age and was given more responsibility when:

Age	Year	Description of Incident

DREAMS

Name:	Age:
Yesterday's Dreams	
Today's Dreams	
How Do I Get There?	
When Should I Get There?	
How Old Was I for Yesterday's Dreams?	
Which Dreams Came True?	
What Dreams Did My Parents Have?	
What Dreams Did My Grandparents Have?	

CHANGE

Name: Age:

Topics: History, Education, Styles, Geography, Politics, Science, Values, Art

Date	Topic	Description of Change	My Reaction

HEROISM/COWARDICE

Name: Age:

Date		
Persons Involved (countries or companies)		
Description of Incident		
Heroism or Cowardice?		

Justification: Justify Your Choice for Heroism or Cowardice for Each of the Incidents You Cited

Heroism	Cowardice

TRIALS AND TRIBULATIONS

Name: Age:

My Trials and Tribulations

Date	Description of Incident	How I Responded
Outcome:		

My Partner's Trials and Tribulations

Date	Description of Incident	His/Her Response
Outcome:		

Trials and Tribulations of Literary Character

Title of Story, Novel, or Poem:
Character's name:

Date	Description of Incident	His/Her Response
Outcome:		

VISIONS

Name: Age:

Story Title:

Character's Name	Description of Vision	Description of Your Vision

Daily Observation Sheet

Name: Age:

Activity Description	Time/Date	Movement Description

Character Observation

Title of Literary Work:

Character's Name:

Activity Description	Time/Date	Movement Description

Annotated Bibliography

The following selected books are excellent resources for either pre-training or working within the nursing home. Ideas for follow-up arts activities follow each synopsis.

ELEMENTARY SCHOOL

Aldridge, J. 1961. *A Penny and a Periwinkle*. Berkeley, Cal.:   Parnassus Press.

The main character is "Old Sy," a fisherman on the coast of Maine. The story compares Sy's simple lifestyle to that of very busy businessmen who come to visit. This is an excellent book for values exploration and the study of careers and geography.

Movement exercise: Explore the arm movements of casting a fishing line. Compare the movements of Sy, who is relaxed, to the very busy men from the big city.

Found Sounds: Compare the sounds of the city with the sounds of the seashore. Divide into two groups and make the sounds.

Climo, Shirley. 1982.   *The Cobweb Christmas*. New York: Thomas Y. Crowell.

A story about a little old woman who receives a special magical gift on Christmas.

Music: Find out if anyone in the nursing home is of German descent. Is anyone in the classroom of German descent? Learn to sing a Christmas carol in German with the senior adults.

Visual Art: Make spider webs out of paper that resemble the ones on Tante's Christmas tree.

Egger, B. 1987. *Marianne's Grandmother.* New York: E.P. Dutton.

A very sensitive book about as little girl whose grandmother has died. It is told through the voice of the child, who expresses some realistic reactions to death such as anger, confusion, and sadness. The book, however, offers positive reinforcement as the child begins to remember of the good things about her grandmother and their relationship. In the end she draws a picture of her grandmother.

Visual Art: Have children draw a picture of their grandmother or grandfather. If they are working with the seniors at the nursing home, have them draw pictures of each other.

Draw pictures of "fun" events you have shared with an older family member.

Oral History: Has your grandmother or grandfather ever told you any funny stories about when she or he was young? Or a story about your mother or father when they were little?

If working with a senior adult: Have your senior adult partner tell you a funny story about when he or she was young. Can you act the story out together?

Goldman, Susan. 1978. 2d printing. *Grandma Is Somebody Special.* Chicago: Albert Whitman and Co.

The narrator goes to visit her "modern" grandmother who has a job and also attends school. The young narrator talks about the special attention the grandmother gives to her.

Oral History: This book is an excellent book to lead into oral history, as in one portion of the book the grandmother tells her grandaughter about a funny event which happened between herself and the child's grandfather.

If read at the nursing home to the intergenerational group, this may help to motivate senior adults to talk about funny incidents in their lives they would like to share with the younger participants.

Younger participants may, at the end of the session, draw a picture for their senior partner or perhaps may send a picture from school. (Receiving correspondence, especially if it's as happy as a child's drawing, is always an uplifting experience.)

Henkes, K. 1986. *Granpa & Bo*. New York: Greenwillow Books.

This book is conducive to intergenerational learning as Bo visits his grandfather in the country and learns various skills. One interesting aspect of this book is that while the grandfather tells Bo stories, Bo also tells the grandfather stories.

Oral History: Youth and senior adult partners should make a chart of hobbies, favorite foods, and likes and dislikes and fill in the chart and compare.

Share a favorite story with each other.

Hoguet, S. 1983. *I Unpacked My Grandmother's Trunk*. New York: E.P. Dutton.

The book is based on a popular word game and includes delightful illustrations. At the beginning of the book are directions for playing the game. The book also encourages children in learning the alphabet. What better way to learn then through a game with senior adults!

Visual Art: Have children ask senior adults what they would pack in a trunk if they had one. Draw illustrations of those items. Perhaps break up the group and assign two or three letters to each group, as using the entire alphabet might be overwhelming.

Lobel, A. 1968. *The Comic Adventures of Old Mother Hubbard and Her Dog.* Englewood Cliffs, N.J.: Bradbury Press.

The book offers the possibility for participation by many different characters as Old Mother Hubbard goes to the baker's, the undertaker's, the fishmonger's, the fruiterer's, and a variety of other places in an effort to make her dog happy.

Creative Drama: Act out each of the scenes as Old Mother Hubbard visits each shop. Discuss the various occupations and what they mean. Also an excellent opportunity for a costume parade.

Rylant, C. 1985. *The Relatives Came.* New York: Bradbury Press.

Relatives pile into a car and make the journey to visit relatives in the mountains. A delightful story to introduce the study of family history and reunions.

Visual Arts: Senior adults and children help each other to draw family trees. Teacher may send home questionnaire sheet with children as a pre-project activity to allow them to continue this in the nursing home. Think about the talents of each relative and draw a picture or symbol beside their name that best represents this flair.

Movement/Music: Study the illustrations in the books. As you can see, there is a great deal of movement, whether it's in the car ride, at the picnic, or even during sleeping. Explore the movement in the book by reproducing it or by giving your own interpretation.

Skorpen, L. 1975. *Mandy's Grandmother*. New York: Dial Press.

For higher elementary or beginning middle school. The book explores a little girl's perception of how a grandmother should be in contrast to what her grandmother really is. The book investigates the relationship between these generations and shows how communication can develop and thus alleviate misunderstandings.

Pre-Project Training: An excellent book to use at both the school and the nursing home in pre-project training. After the book has been read, the following questions might be asked:

1. What kinds of things do you do with your grandmother or grandfather?

2. What kinds of things would you like to do with your grandmother or grandfather? (If the child does not have regular contact with grandparents or does not have grandparents rephrase question as a "What if."

3. What happened in the story to make Mandy change her mind about her grandmother?

4. Why do you think Mandy's grandmother changed her mind about her grandaughter?

5. Make a list of the way Mandy and her grandmother are alike.

6. Make a list of how they are different.

7. Make a list of how you are like your grandmother or grandfather.

8. Make a list of how you are different.

The same questions might be asked at the nursing home, but from the viewpoint of the senior adult.

Stevenson, James. 1983. *Granpa's Great City Tour*. New York: Green Willow
      Books.

     An alphabet book for children where a grandfather takes them on a
tour of a city.

Visual Arts: If your grandmother or grandfather came to school with you,
what would you show them? Find something in the room that begins with the
letter "A." (The teacher may have set out objects that children may find or they
may delightedly find objects of their own.) Can you draw a picture of the
object?

Williams, B. 1975. *Kevin's Grandma*. New York: E.P. Dutton.

     A delightful book which compares two very different grandmothers,
one very modern and one very traditional.

Pre-training: Used in the nursing home, ask each resident to describe
themselves in comparison to the book. Would they be considered traditional
or modern? One interesting response in the past has been, "I would probably
be considered traditional, but just once, I'd like to be modern!"

     In school, after reading the book, have each student make a list of
characteristics of each of the grandmothers in the story. Have students make a
third column and describe their own grandmother or grandfather.

     What will they be like when they are old?

MIDDLE AND HIGH SCHOOL

Novels

Source: "Charles Dickens' Old People." D. Charles and L. Charles. 1979-80
      International Journal of Aging and Human Development 10 (3): pp.
      231-37.

Charles Dickens's Characters: In a study conducted by Don and Linda Charles (1979-80) in which more than 120 of Charles Dickens's characters were examined, it was reported that "Dickens' old people were fully engaged in life and society and were not age-segregated" (p.231). In fact, "Charles Dickens was an exception to the rule of literary neglect of old characters"(p.232). Furthermore, in studying the novels they found that the older characters most often appeared in supporting rather than leading roles. Some of the most intriguing and well-defined characters, however, are those who play supporting roles. They appear quickly and affect the major character's life. Because they appear for a short time, it is important that their portraits be complete, and therefore the literary painting of such characters is very important. For theater students, study of such supporting roles is important, to look further for stage interpretation of these roles. Many times, students of drama and literature have a tendency to ignore the importance of supporting or minor characters. It is the minor characters, however, who help to move the action along and force major characters to make decisions. For this reason, the works of Dickens should be studied for both the minor and major character influences, especially intergenerational ones. In studying minor characters, students become involved in a more intricate and finite study of the novel. The use of a "web" (see chart, Appendix B) might help in organizing thoughts and present a fine visual indication of the process of major character and minor character support. Some works of Dickens that might be included in the middle and high school curriculum are *David Copperfield, A Christmas Carol, Great Expectations, A Tale of Two Cities*, and *Oliver Twist*.

Activities

1. **Review:** Students and nursing home residents present a review of particular scenes that involve intergenerational themes. Residents might help youngsters review for a test by drawing the names of minor characters from a hat and asking students to describe how the minor character affected the life of a major character.

2. **Dramatization:** Present dramatizations of particular passages that involve intergenerational exchanges.

Discuss the impact of the older character upon the younger one and vice versa.

3. Age-Search: Students might also engage in a "search-for-the-young" and "search-for-the-old" in literary works with a reading/library group at the nursing home. Those studying Dickens's older characters will be interested in the Charleses' findings that it "was not unusual to discover that an old-acting character was in his thirties or a young-acting character much older than first assumed" (p.236).   Participants and students involved in the study will have to pay particular attention to the information in order to win the search game.

4. Character Study: The Charleses' findings futhermore state that the "Dickens people are *persons* first, and only incidentally persons of a particular age" (p.236). Students and residents might discuss and chart the personality traits of each of the characters in the novel.

5. Visual Arts: Students and residents should study the "Sketches By Boz" and examine costume, character relationships, "visual attitudes," and artistic style.

Zindel, Paul. 1986. *The Pigman*. New York: Bantam Books.
Zindel, Paul. 1988. *The Pigman's Legacy*. New York: Bantam Books.

Both Zindel books involve the escapades of two young people, Lorraine Jensen and John Conlan, with elderly men.   These books are especially good for high interest/low motivation readers and may be shared in a reading group with residents at a nursing home. They are also appropriate for pre-training at either site as they present clear pictures of contemporary adolescents and the elderly.

Poetry

Maclay, Elsie, ed. 1977. *Green Winter: Celebrations of Old Age.* New York: Thomas Y. Crowell.

One volume of poetry worth studying in its entirety is that of *Green Winter: Celebrations of Old Age*, edited by Elsie Maclay. "The word portraits in this book are of real people. But they are not interviews. They are reflections of the spirit of men and women I have known..."(p. xiii).

This book is divided into sections, the first of which is "Assessing and Defining."

Activities

"My Children Are Coming Today": This selection might be used in studying the question of independence. In the poem, an older person compares her adult children's hesitancy in leaving her alone to her hesitancy as a mother in leaving her children alone. This reflective poem might be used in discussing and comparing independence for the young adult and the elderly. Why is the feeling of independence so crucial for the young adult? Why is it important when you're older?

"Teacher": For teachers, this poem which explores the absence due to illness of a teacher in her seventies from class poses an interesting idea. When the instructor returns, her students' response is

> Look what we did without you -
> This and this and this -
> We don't need you!
> to which the teacher replies,
> 'That's wonderful.
> You know, that's the nicest thing a
> Teacher can hear.
> I'm proud to know
> I taught you so well you can go on
> Without me.' (p. 6)

This might even be interesting with students responding and offering a new insight into student-teacher relationships.

"Dreams": Yet another moment of sharing is offered through the poem "Dreams," which may lead to a cross-generational experience as the elderly share their dreams of the past with youth who share their dreams of the future. The youth might also help the elderly to come up with new dreams. This exercise might also serve as a life review technique as both ages reminisce about dreams of the past. The activity might also be expanded into an organizational life plan for expressing and reviewing dreams and then organizing goals and plans for implementation (see chart, Appendix B). At the end of the poem, the author is asking for an opportunity for one or two dreams, which might be a good stimulus for discussion. Envisioning dreams may be a first step in the study of self-actualization, a healthy activity no matter what one's age or financial/societal background.

"Shaving": For the male adolescent, the poem "Shaving" (p.20) offers insight into future years of grooming. Discussion concerning "rites of passage" may follow for both male and female participants. An interesting question for the youth to ask is what was the first grown-up privilege your parents allowed you? This might also help the youth to stand once removed from their own personal longing and struggle for adulthood as they hear about the experiences of others. (Also see chart, Appendix B, for "Rites of Passage.")

"This Changing World": An absolutely delightful poem for all ages is "This Changing World." This particular poetic reflection gives the reader a new insight into change. It is of especial interest to the youth of today as they will witness incredible change over the next decade. Our elderly have lived through the rapidity of change our youth will be faced with. Thus, the reading and subsequent discussion of this poem might lead to interesting insights into dealing with change. (See chart for mapping of change, Appendix B.)

"Grandchildren": Under the heading of "The Courage of Friends" comes the poem "Grandchildren" (p.86). In it, the author praises children and youth even while their parents are disappointed. It is yet another excellent avenue for discussion and for making a positive link between the generations. Through the thoughts of this poem, the youth are able to see their own value, whereas adults might reprimand their behavior and the elderly see beyond.

"Baskets": This poem (p.106) offers humor mixed with history as an older woman imagines the impact of homemade baskets across the ages and cultures. The poem has an amusing anecdote as the writer talks about her eighteen year-old granddaughter "Writing from her fancy Eastern college: 'I'm taking a course in basketry'" (p.106). Students may find two levels of discussion here: one concerning the cultures mentioned in the poem, the Egyptians, Mayans, Hungarians, and Sioux and what we may learn from these cultures and the other concerning what may be passed down from generation to generation.

"Our Secret": This poem attests to the fun of being old. Both groups could benefit from making a chart listing the advantages of being old and those of being young. It is interesting that the poem lists some things that are equally appealing to elderly and youth alike. Such things as: "The world gets off your back," "Watching a spider spin a web," "eating applesauce and cream instead of dinner," "dawdling," and "staying up all night" (p.123) reach across the generations as clearly as some lightning bolts stretch across the sky.

"Old Lovers":   Another common subject of interest is
love. In the poem "Old Lovers" (p.128), the author not
only reminds us that love can happen at any age but also
pinpoints some of the feelings of love. This poem,
combined with the study of the one-act play, *A Sunny
Morning* (Serafin and Joaquin Alvarez Quintero), places
both couples on park benches at the opening of their
scenarios. Discussions of how various residents met and
courted or were courted by their spouses may follow. A
comparative chart exploring the similarities and
differences in dating customs lends an interesting
ambiance to the gathering.

Plays

Alvarez Quintero, Serafin and Joaquin.   1984.   *A Sunny Morning*. In
       Understanding Literature.   New York: Macmillan Publishing
       Company.

While the play concerns the reuniting of an elderly couple, it also
compares youthful love with older love. This can be used very effectively at the
high school level and at the nursing home. Responses of residents, after the
reading and dramatization of the play at the nursing home, to the question,
"What is love?" included the following:

    1) good friendship, 2) kindness, 3) deepest friendship
    between two people, 4) caring, 5) happy, 6) smile, 7)
    deep love grows slow, 8) learn to shake hands and make
    up, 9) if you fall out, make up.

    Interestingly enough, the responses of the young
    people were the same with one or two added items:

    1) someone who cares about you, and 2) you know
    you have a date for the prom! (Clark 1988)

Diggs, Elizabeth. 1981. *Close Ties*. New York: Nelson Doubleday, Inc.

    *Due to some subject matter and language, parental permission might
be needed for public school study.

The play takes place in the Frye summer house in the Berkshires where members of the family gather. The central focus of the play concerns the decision to commit the eighty-four year old grandmother to a nursing home. The play illustrates the difficulties in making such a decision and the impact of the differing opinions upon the family.

Activities

1. Participants should read the description of the kitchen, (p.3), and discuss changes in design. Attention should be given to the combination of the old and the young in this particluar room of the house.

2. Participants should discuss Josephine's advice regarding marriage (p.23).

3. Participants should discuss Josephine's views regarding old age (pp. 25, 77).

4. Participants should discuss Watt's and Bess's ideas concerning nursing homes (p.47).

5. Participants should discuss Joesphine's long-term memory (p.77). What incidents does she recall?

6. Participants should discuss each character's reaction to placing Josephine at Millbrook and consider whether or not they agree with the final decision.

Noss, Elyse. 1990. *Three One-Act Plays About the Elderly.* New York: Samuel French, Inc.

The three plays included in this collection, *The Cat Connection, Second Chance,* and *Admit One,* may be used for pre-training, scene study and discussion, and/or production.

Second Chance

Through the study of this play, participants may compare two very different philosophies of life expressed by two older women.

Activities

1. After reading the play, participants should compare Rita's approach to life with Evelyn's approach. Participants should discuss which lifestyle they themselves prefer.

2. Participants should discuss Evelyn's dream to become a painter, (p.21), and live in Paris. Participants should also fill out the Dreams worksheet together (Appendix B).

3. Participants should discuss the characters' differing opinions concerning exercise.

4. Participants should discuss whether or not they feel Evelyn will change after seeing Rita's play.

Admit One

This one-act presents an interesting study of the relationship between seventy-five year old Harold Conklin and fifty-nine year old Megan Matthews. Harold has placed an advertisement for a female companion in the newspaper to which Megan has responded.

Activities

1. After reading the play, participants should discuss the changes Harold talks about, (p.51), and use the Changes worksheet, (Appendix B), to list additional changes.

2. Discuss whether or not the minsunderstanding between these two characters is age-related.

The Cat Connection

This one-act offers the reader an insight into two different older women, May Reynolds and Leona Woods, who are both in their late sixties. The play concerns their meeting on a park bench and feeding a cat. As the play progresses, we learn more about each character's trials and tribulations.

Activities

1. After reading the play, participants should fill in the
Trails and Tribulations worksheet (Appendix B).

2. Participants should discuss past illnesses and
remedies. Youth partners and elderly participants may
make a list of old-fashioned remedies.

3. Participants should discuss how friendship develops
between these two women. A further discussion might
include friends of the youth and elderly partners and
how those relationships developed.

4. Participants should consider whether this play could
be about any age.

Osborn, Paul. 1967. *Morning's At Seven*. Garrden City, New York: Nelson
    Doubleday, Inc.

This play, about the lives of four elderly sisters and their families, was
originally produced in 1939. It offers the reader an opportunity to study family
crisis and resolution.

Activities

1. After reading the play, participants should compare
the social impact of this play during the 1930s to the
social impact it might have today. Discuss how the
public's view of the older woman may have changed.

2. Participants should discuss references made to aging
by the following characters: Myrtle (p.22), Homer
(p.25), Ida (p.35), David (p.53), Thor (p.80), Esther
(p.100), and Aary (p.136).

3. Participants should discuss Esther's feelings that she
can now be "free." Consider if this has changed for
today's grandmother. Consider how it might change in
the future.

4. Participants should discuss Homer's relationship with his mother and with Myrtle. How do these relationships add further complications to the plot?

5. Participants should make a list of "old-fashioned" names and discuss why certain names are popular during different periods in history. Participants should think of names in their family. Which ones are considered "old-fashioned" and which ones are modern? Consider why each child was given a particular name.

6. It seems that each one of these characters comes to an awakening. Participants should discuss each character's experience of awakening. Participants should consider one of the myths of aging that "old people are incapable of change."

7. Participants should discuss the characters' views of marriage (pp.149-150) and consider how these opinions may have changed since the 1920s.

8. Although this play is about older people, the action takes on an accelerated pace as soon as Carl begins to help David with the bathroom. Participants should discuss the pacing of the play and the number of events which take place.

Redgrave, Michael. 1959. *The Aspern Papers*. Adpated from the short story by Henry James. New York: Samuel French, Inc.

Henry, James. 1888. "The Aspern Papers." In *Henry James Selected Fiction*. Leon Edel, ed. New York: E. P. Dutton and Company, 1964.

Participants should read both the novelette and the play adaptation and compare the two. Both concern the experiences of a writer, Henry Jarvis (H. J.), as he attempts to secure personal papers for a book he is researching. His relationships with the elderly Miss Julianna Bordereau and her niece, Tina, as he attempts to gain their confidence, add further intrigue to this interesting study of human behavior.

Activities

1. While H. J. is trying to convince Tina to rent a room
to him, he talks about the value of European history as
compared to that of America. Participants should study
the passage from the play, (p.15), and discuss H. J.'s
insights regarding Europe and America.

2. Participants should discuss how Miss Julianna feels
about living as described by her niece, Tina (p.24). Is
this a feeling which is common among the elderly?

3. Participants should study Tina's dialogue regarding
gentleman of the past and present (p.47). Younger
participants might ask older participants to list criteria
for gentleman of the past. The two groups may then
compare ideas concerning the definition of a gentleman.

4. Participants should study Miss Julianna's actions as
she relishess the past (p.51). What event does she seem
to be reliving?

Wright, William A., ed. 1936. *The Complete Works of Shakespeare*. New
York: Doubleday, Inc.

Draper, John W. 1946. "Shakespeare's Attitude Towards Old People." *Journal
of Gerontology* 1:118-126.

An interesting assignment for participants to explore is the study of
older characters in Shakespeare's plays and their influence upon younger
characters. Although "aged" during Elizabethan times was younger than our
present day chronological definition, the ensuing relationships are worth
examination. Also worth investigation is a comprehensive study of
Shakespeare's changing views of aging (Draper 1946).

Activities

Romeo and Juliet

Act I, scene iii - A room in Capulet's house

1. Participants should consider what reflections the nurse offers to Juliet in regards to men.

2. How is the Nurse portrayed in this scene?

Act II, scene iii - Friar Laurence's cell

1. What advice does the Friar give to Romeo regarding love? Do you agree or disagree with this advice? Younger participants should ask their elderly partners for advice they might give concerning the topic of love.

Act II, scene iv - A street

1. Describe Benvolio and Mercutio's treatment of the Nurse. Compare their treatment of her with the treatment of the elderly in today's society.

Act II, scene v - Capulets's orchard

1. Find and discuss Juliet's description of older people. Do you agree or disagree with her view?

Act III, scene ii - Capulet's orchard

1. Find and discuss the Nurse's reference to being old.

King Lear

Act I, scene i - King Lear's Palace

1. Discuss Goneril's explanation concerning changes brought about by the aging process.

Act I, scene ii - The Earl of Gloucester's Castle

1. Discuss the contents of the letter read by Gloucester. What references are made to the aging process?

2. Discuss Edmund's philosophy concerning sons and their aging fathers.

Act I, scene iii - The Duke of Albany's Palace

1. Discuss Goneril's statement concerning old fools.

Act III, scene iii - Gloucester's Castle

1. Discuss Edmund's statement concerning the rise of the young and the fall of the old.

Act III, scene vi - A chamber in a farmhouse adjoining the castle

1. Discuss Lear's mock trial of his daughters. Is he mental imbalance due to age or circumstance?

Act IV, scene vi - Fields near Dover

1. Discuss Lear's attire as he enters. A visual arts activity might be to sketch what this costume would look like and compare renderings.

Act IV, scene vii - A tent in the French camp

1. Discuss Lear's description of himself as an old man.

Act V, scene iii - The British Camp near Dover

1. Discuss Albany's statement regarding the old and the young.

Short Stories

Crane, Stephen. 1963. "The Veteran." In *The Complete Stories and Sketches of Stephen Crane*. Thomas A. Gullason, ed. New York: Doubleday, Inc.

The story opens with Henry Fleming telling tales of war in the grocery store. The conversation comes around to a point of discussion concerning war. We watch and listen as a grandson's vision of his grandfather as a war hero is shattered only to be redefined through the grandfather's valor and heroism in saving animals from a barnyard fire.

This story offers the adolescent the opportunity to examine heroism and cowardice and to study the true definition of valor. In light of the events taking place in the year 1990, this study of heroism during wartime is especially relevant.

Activities

1. Students may ask themselves in which war did Henry Fleming participate and compare it to the Vietnam War, or to any current boundary and power dispute of today.

2. Students may look at the changing relationship between Henry Fleming and his grandson Jimmy. Of especial consideration might be the following description:

When little Jim walked with his grandfather he was in the habit of skipping along on the stone pavement in front of the three stores and the hotel of the town and betting that he could avoid the cracks. But upon this day he walked soberly, with his hand gripping two of his grandfather's fingers. Sometimes he kicked abstractly at dandelions that curved over the walk. Anyone could see that he was much troubled. (p.292)

The story then takes a turn, as one of the hired men gets drunk and overturns his lantern in the barn. Only the old man is brave enough to run into the fire to try to save the horses and cows.

3. At this point, it might be helpful for students to study the story's literary images, which are especially enchanting in the last paragraph:

When the roof fell in, a great funnel of smoke swarmed toward the sky, as if the old man's mighty spirit, released from its body - a little bottle - had swelled like the genie of fable. The smoke was tinted rose-hue from the flames, and perhaps the unutterable midnights of the universe will have no power to daunt the color of his soul. (p.294)

Students might work with art classes to illustrate this final passage, as the visual imagry is strong and compelling.

4. Students may make a chart, with social studies and history classes, that lists various wars and examples of heroism and cowardice (see chart, Appendix B.)

Taylor, Peter.   1969. "Miss Leonora When Last Seen." In *The Collected Stories Of Peter Taylor*. New York: Farrar, Straus, and Giroux.

The story, which takes place in Thomasville, concerns the disappearance of Miss Leonora Logan, a retired teacher. We find out at the beginning that she has been missing for two weeks, having left on her own accord driving a 1942 Dodge convertible.
The reason for her disappearance is stated as follows:

The cause of all our present tribulation is this: The Logan property, which Miss Leonora inherited from one of her paternal great-uncles and which normally upon her death would have gone to distant relatives of hers in Chicago, has been chosen as a site for our county's new consolidated high school. (p.504)

The story traces the history of Miss Leonora's teaching career, highlighting some of the major events in a town faced with gradual urbanization. Because it is told through the heart and voice of one of her former pupils, now a grown man, we find an interesting sentiment mixed with maturity.

Miss Leonora's motivation for taking these trips was always, until the present instance, something that that it even seemed pointless to speculate on.. ..But if anything happens to her now, all the world will blame *us* and say we *sent* her on this journey, sent her out alone and possibly in a dangerous frame of mind. In particular, the blame will fall on the four timid male citizens who were the last in Thomasville (for I do not honestly believe we will ever see her alive again) and who, as old friends and former pupils of hers at the high school ought to have prevented her going away. (pp.505-06)

Part II of the story weaves us in and out of integration and gives a more detailed history of the Logan family. Part III begins with Miss Leonora's house being condemned and takes us through the repercussions.

Activities

1. Because the story describes various mannerisms of Miss Leonora, it might be interesting for students to list and describe the mannerisms of their various teachers. The elderly may remember mannerisms of their former teachers. In actor training this type of exercise proves invaluable as students must study their own physical habits as well as those of others in order to portray effectively an array of characters.

2. Students might share discussions with older people about their favorite teacher and their least favorite teacher.

3. Students should discuss the definition of growth within a town or city. Refer to page 507, which tells about the history of the Logan family beginning with the Civil War and how the family may have impeded the growth of the town. Are these things really growth?

4. Part III begins with Miss Leonora's house being condemned and the subsequent change in Miss Leonora's style. Students should discuss the change in Miss Leonora and study the following passages from the story:

"You may be too late," Buck added as I was turning away. I looked back at him with lifted eyebrows. "She was in here a while ago," he went on to report, "getting her car gassed up. She said how she was about to take off on one of her trips. She said she might wait till she heard from the courthouse this afternoon and again she might not.. ..She was got up kind of peculiar." (p. 527)

I saw at a glance that this wasn't the Miss Leonora I had known, and wasn't one that I had heard about from her tourist-home friends, either. (p. 530)

The story describes in detail how much she has changed and portrays her leaving. Students should discuss change in people and the myth that old people are incapable of change.

5. Students should study the last passage in the story:

The postcards she sends us indicate nothing about how she is dressed, of course, or about where and in what kind of places she is stopping. She says only that she is in good health, that it is wonderful weather for driving about the country, and that the roads have been improved everywhere. She says nothing about when we can expect her to come home. (p. 533)

Why is the last sentence so haunting? The author endears this woman to us but in a realistic manner so that we see her as a human being, with all the idiosyncracies of human nature. We know what she was about without his ever having discussed her as a child. At the end, we share the author's haunting sense of sadness that Miss Leonora may never return. Students should consider the following questions: Has this ever happened to you? Have you had to leave a place or has someone you cared about ever had to leave? How did you feel about your departure or their absence?

6. Students should draw a life graph for Miss Leonora. Try to incorporate some of the high points in her life as well as the low points.

7. Students should compare the town of Thomasville to the town in which they live. They should ask the elderly about the characteristics of the small hometown. Perhaps theirs is like the one in the story. Students should consider how their town has changed.

8. Students should look at a map and together with an elderly person, chart her travels. They should consider how these places have changed.

9. Students should consider how education has changed since Miss Leonora taught.

10. Students should write a profile of their most memorable teacher. Have their elderly partner do the same. Partners should compare their impressions and memories.

Welty, Eudora. 1974. "A Worn Path" In *The Art of Fiction*. R. F. Dietrich, and R. H. Sundell, eds. New York: Holt Rinehart and Winston.

This short story becomes an excellent study of characterization as we travel along with the elderly Phoenix Jackson on her journey on foot to obtain medicine.

Activities

1. When this story was shared with a reading/library group in South Boston, Virginia, a reaction of elderlyparticipants was that the trials and tribulations they faced in life were comparable to those of Phoenix Jackson as she goes through in the woods and town to reach her destination. Students may want to

compare their journeys through life with the journey of Phoenix Jackson (see chart, Appendix B).

2. This particular story has been dramatized in theatre classes at the high school and at the nursing home with great success.

3. Phoenix presents an excellent opportunity for character study.

4. The story presents an excellent opportunity for the study of costume design. Students should pay particular attention to the description of Phoenix at the beginning of the story.

Thomas, Dylan. 1970. "A Visit to Grandpa's." In *Vision and Value: A Thematic Introduction to the Short Story*. James Nagel, ed. Belmont, Cal.: Dickenson Publishing Company.

This particular story is advisable only for advanced high school students, as there is strong material with the possible suicide of the grandfather at the end of the story.

Activities

1. Students may engage in serious discussions regarding the old man's suicide. Students may also investigate current statistics regarding teenage and elderly suicide.

2. Students should list the activities and places the narrator and his grandfather visited. Students should consider the following questions: Do you have grandparents or memories of what you did together?

3. The teacher might pose the following challenge: Compare your placing a pair of headphones on your head, turning up your stereo, and singing at the top of your lungs to Grandpa's "midnight rides" in the story.

4. Students should consider why the old man might be ready to die.

5. Students should consider the last sentence: "But Grandpa stood firmly on the bridge, and clutched his bag to his side, stared at the flowing river and the sky, like a prophet who has no doubt" (p. 340).

Students should compare this paragraph with the last paragraph in "The Veteran" by Stephen Crane. They should illustrate the last paragraph and compare this artwork with artwork from "The Veteran."

6. Students should compare what the young man in "The Veteran" learned about his grandfather with the young man's findings in this story.

Adonjan, Carol. 1981. "The Room With the View." *North American Review* (March):25-27.

This short story is advisable only for advanced high school students because it contains mature subject matter. Through the telling of this story, we live through the daily events of a middle-aged woman and her elderly mother who, through circumstance, have come to live together in the same house.

The reader, having been exposed to the visions of both characters, comes away with a new vision for life and the process of dying.

Activities

1. Study the passage concerning the cut- glass bowl: "(she saw one exactly like it in an antique store window just the other day: one hundred and twenty-five dollars)" (p. 26).

Discuss antique cut-glass bowls--Why are they so valuable today? Students should combine with art classes to study this particular era of art. Students should also discuss with the residents popular designs of their era and find illustrations that exhibit these designs.

2. Students and residents should engage in a discussion regarding vision. What does the Old Woman see that the younger woman, her daughter, fails to see? Make a chart to illustrate their separate visions.

3. Discuss the following passage:

She sits motionless before the windows, her eyes fixed in such a way that she appears to her daughter to be looking inward, studying some secret interior landscape. And she does not report the things she has seen. She says only, "This is a lovely room. I have always liked a room with a view!" (p. 27)

Visual Art Assignment: Create a "vision painting" that illustrates either your visions or the visions of the characters in the story.

Photography Assignment: Travel around the nursing home with your elderly partner. Take pictures looking out from various windows. If possible take pictures from the outside looking in as well. Develop the photographs and discuss the various visions you and your partner discovered.

Lamb, Margaret. 1970. "Management" In *Women on Woman Alone*. 1977. L. Hamalian and L. Hamalian, eds. New York: Delacorte Press.

This story concerns the trials and tribulations of elderly Bitsy Larkin as she tries to survive on a fixed income. The story presents an interesting example not only of the of economics of old age, but of relationships and inner strength.

Activities

1. Study the following passage:

No one knows how old she is. Bitsy was never told the year she was born, only that it was in freedom.

Despite the sun and her sweaters, she shivers. She
is so old and thin that she is always cold, and holds her
arms tight across her wishbone chest. Her nose and
chin, once sharp, are fallen, but she holds her neck stiff.
(p. 25)

Students should pay particular attention to the
descriptive writing here. A visual art assignment might
be to create a pen-and-ink study of the main character.

2. Study the following passage:

Bitsy always goes straight home from the bank,to put
aside the rent money. This way there is never the
danger of being put out--or of having to ask the welfare
for more money. Many people she knows cannot live on
their check; they eat the rent, and then the landlord
wants his room. But Bitsy eats less as she gets older.
She is always very careful in her spending, and so she
gets along. (p. 26)

Students should become familiar with Social
Security and Medicare benefits and what is entailed in
living on a fixed income. They might engage in
discussions with elderly residents and inquire about
struggles, ideas for saving, and shortcuts, as were
discovered by the main character in this story.

3. Bitsy is attacked and her money stolen. The
second time this happens, her landlady, Mrs. Frazer,
takes her down to the welfare office and suggests she be
placed in a nursing home. Discuss Bitsy's reaction to
being placed in a nursing home.

4. A man "comes to her rescue"--so she thinks. He
takes her money for "moving expenses," and Bitsy must
return to welfare to request additional funds for "added
expenses."
Two characters share an understanding by the end
of the story, as Bitsy has become both business- and

street- smart. The man has learned that perhaps Bitsy is not as "dumb" as she looks. It appears that they may work together to survive.

Students should discuss the lessons Bitsy learned and the importance of business sense and street sense.

Pingwa, Jia. trans. by Hu Zbibui. 1987. "Shasha and the Pigeons." *Short Story International*, 2(65):37-50.

The story opens with a boy with his head shaved peering at a man who keeps pigeons. As the boy gains the trust of the man, a relationship develops that is important not only to the two characters but eventually to the entire town.

Activities

1. This story gives students a perfect opportunity to study Asian art. Read and study the following excerpt and illustrate the passage: "In the lane, only I kept pigeons, twelve all. Of various colors--red, black, white, and spotted--they were all perched on the earthen wall in a row just under the eaves of my house." (p.37)

2. We find out that the boy comes from a broken home and lives with his father in order to have a better opportunity for future employment. We also learn that the mother lives in the country and is taking care of the grandfather.

"No, Grandpa doesn't want her to go away, so she's still at home. She said she would look after Grandpa until his death." (p. 39)

Discuss what the boy's relationship might be with his grandfather.

3. Study the following passage from the story and discuss what linking forces in friendships you might have with others.

"I had never thought that he could be so animated and humorous. In ten days, he told me a lot of similar anecdotes. For my part, I taught him in return about raising pigeons. In this way, we soon became bosom friends." (p. 41)

4. Shasha's father forbids him to come to see the man and his pigeons. Students should discuss loneliness or the loss of a friend with their elderly partner. Unfortunately, the death of a friend has become a linking force between the elderly and youth of today as both are faced with with life-threatening diseases regardless of age. "As little Shasha couldn't come any more, I sat reading in the courtyard feeling very lonely" (p.43).

Cormier, Robert. 1983. "The Moustache." In *Best Short Stories*. Raymond Harris, ed. Providence, R.I.: Jamestown Publishers.

Mike's grandmother suffers from arteriosclerosis. When he goes to the nursing home to visit her, she mistakes him for her deceased husband. His presence and moustache (even the way he is dressed) prompt the grandmother's long-term memory as she reminisces, particularly about the time her husband bought a grand piano during the Depression. The most important memory of an incident, however, involves a time when the grandmother placed blame upon her husband in regard to another woman.

In the story, Mike learns a lesson about life from his grandmother and, based on this experience, asks his parents an important question when he comes home.

The book gives the reader many useful activities involving the study of the elderly. For example, the following questions are posed to the reader:

1. How has Mike's grandmother changed from the way she was before she became ill? How does this make you feel about aging?
2. What kind of thoughts are running through Mike's mind as he nears the nursing home?
3. In the course of his visit with his grandmother, what does Mike learn that changes his image of old people in general?

4. What feeling prompts Mike to kiss his grandmother?
(p. 199)

Activities

1. The text shows a drawing of a young man with a moustache looking at an old woman and asks the student to look at the illustration and determine the feelings of the people in the picture.

Visual Art Activity: Students should combine with the art classes and study self-portraits and snapshots of their grandparents.

In the nursing home, students should compare photographs with the photographs of the elderly when they were young.

This activity also presents a perfect opportunity for studying character and old-age makeup.

Slide Show Drama: Take slides of the photographs of the elderly and prepare an oral history script based on the slides. Use the slides as each story is dramatized.

Character-Story Creation: Before students meet their elderly persons, show slides of the individual elderly at the school and allow the students to write a "Fantasy biographical sketch" and a short story based on the slides. Repeat at the nursing homes, using slides of the youth. When the groups meet, have them trade stories.

2. Although arteriosclerosis is defined in the story, students should continue research on this topic. Students should also research long-term and short-term memory.

The activities that follow the story focus upon themes and feelings and ask important questions concerning aging and nursing homes.

Fitzgerald, Francis Scott. 1920. "Bernice Bobs Her Hair." 1957. In *Stories*.
        Frank G. Jennings and Charles J. Calitri, eds.   New York:
        Harcourt, Brace and World, Inc.

This short story concerns the coming of age, centered around a visiting cousin, Bernice, who eventually "bobs" her hair to prove a point. The intergenerational focal point becomes the term"bobbing."

Activities

1. In the nursing home, we read the story and then discussed the term "bob."   Some reactions of the residents when asked, "Did you ever bob your hair?" were as follows: "My mother was mad!" "My boyfriend liked it." "I had hair all the way down to my waist and then I got it bobbed. Everybody was shocked." Most high school students were unfamiliar with the term.

2. Drama classes at school and at the nursing home enjoy dramatizing this story. It also presents an opportunity for comparing hairstyles of the different ages. It is especially appropriate for high schools that have technical training centers for cosmetology.

West, Jessamyn. 1984 "Sixteen." In *Understanding Literature*. New York:
        Macmillan Publishing Company

This story concerns Cress Delahanty, who is at college having a wonderful time when she is unexpectedly summoned home by her parents. The reason is unpleasant since her grandfather is dying. She finds out, however, through an exchange with her grandfather, that she is very much like her grandmother in her love for flowers.
        This, too, is a coming-of-age story in which a young girl learns an important lesson through her infirm grandfather.

Activities

1. Flowers brighten any day for a person, regardless of age! Students should take flowers to the nursing home and read the story with the residents.

2. Students should conduct research pertaining to violets and illustrate various flowers. This might also be done as a collaborative project at the nursing home.

3. As a writing exercise, the elderly and their youth-partners should compare how they are like their grandparents.

4. As a writing or discussion exercise, both groups should consider important life-lessons they may have learned from their grandparents. This could also be extended into lessons the residents could pass on to the students. If there is a school newspaper and a newsletter at the nursing home, both groups might consider trading advice in an ongoing column.

Miscellaneous Listings

Portraits and Pathways : *Discovery Through The Humanities: Exploring Stories of Aging* . 1988. Edited by Jane Deren, Ph.D., with assistance from Ronald J. Manheimer, Ph.D., and Sylvia Riggs Liroff. Discovery Through the Humanities Program in cooperation with The National Center for Health Promotion and Aging. The National Council on the Aging. Washington, D.C.

This large-print collection of prose and poetry, which explores various aspects of aging, is divided into five sections including "Images of Self," "Images of Relationships," "Images of Change," "Images of Creativity," and "Images of Affirmation." This collection also contains photographs by older artists at the beginning of each section and asks the reader reflective questions concerning each photographic study or composition. Each author is given a short autobiographical sketch. This sensitive collection also lends itself to an international flair.

The accompanying *Discussion Leader's Guide* is helpful in curriculum and program planning as it provides the teacher/leader with questions and ideas for thought that are pertinent to each section.

Some particular notes of interest pertaining to intergenerational literature are as follows:

      1."The Measure of My Days" by Florida Scott-Maxwell.

This journal entry sounds almost like the self-reflection of adolescence. A review by high school students and identification of shared feelings with the author might be very helpful in writing their own self-reflections.

      2. "Song" by Adrienne Rich

This poem would be helpful in teaching images and in engaging in discussions about loneliness.

Tisdale, S. 1987. *Harvest Moon: Portrait of a Nursing Home.* New York: Henry Holt Company.

This collection of memories about working in a nursing home is excellent for pre-training at the high school.

Weaver, Frances *The Girls With the Grandmother Faces.* 1987. Colorado Springs,: Century One Press.

This collection of advice, thoughts, stories, and memories is a must for young girls or for any age for that matter. Although the primary audience might be women over fifty-five, Frances Weaver offers the opportunity to readers of any age and gender the time to reflect upon the value of living.

This book might be read in an intergenerational setting and may be used for motivation for the elderly and the youth to write their own reflections. The author also includes a very helpful section, "Now about Writing..." that should encourage and assist any group in writing.

Bibliography

Allard, H. 1977. *It's So Nice to Have a Wolf around the House*. New York: Doubleday and Company.

Allen, M. 1986. "Channel One: An Intergenerational Program at Work." *Children Today* 15 (3):32-34.

Alvarez Quintero, S., and J. Quintero. 1920. "A Sunny Day" In *Understanding Literature*. 1984. New York: Macmillan.

Auden, W.H., L .and Kronenberger. 1981. *Aphorisms*. New York: Penguin Books.

Balkema, John B. 1986. *The Creative Spirit: An Annotated Bibliography on the Arts, Humanities and Aging*. Washington, D.C.: National Council on the Aging.

Barlow, W. 1973. *The Alexander Technique*. New York: Alfred A. Knopf.

Bausell, R., A. Rooney, and C. Inlander. 1988. *How to Evaluate and Select a Nursing Home*. New York: Addison-Wesley Publishing Company.

Berkson, J., and S. Griggs. 1986. "An Intergenerational Program at a Middle School." *The School Counselor* 34:140-43.

Blake, G. 1986. "Project MAIN: Classwork in the Community Benefits Senior Citizens." *Children Today* 15 (4):31-34.

Bottum, D. (producer/director), J. Metal-Corbin, G. Barker (project directors), and D. Corbin (narrator/writer). 1985. *Age Doesn't Matter: Weaving Dance and Aging into a Fifth Grade Curriculum*. Videotape. Omaha: University Television, University of Nebraska at Omaha.

Bowers, D. 1976. "Ethiopia." George Mason University publication.

Buck, P. "The Good Deed." 1953. In *Understanding Literature* 1984. New York: Macmillan.

Caplow-Lindner. 1979. *Therapeutic Dance Movement: Expressive Activities for Older Adults*. New York: Human Sciences Press.

Cardosi, J. 1982. "I Remember How My Mother Used to Hold Me, God: A Look at Touching the Elderly." Paper presented at the Virginia Speech Communication Association, Rhetoric and Communication Theory Division, October.

Cetron, M., B. Soriano, and M. Gale. 1985. *Schools of the Future: How American Business Can Cooperate to Save Our Schools*. New York: McGraw-Hill Book Company.

Clark, M. 1980. "The Poetry of Aging: Views of Old Age in Contemporary American Poetry." *The Gerontologist* 20:188-91.

Clark, P. 1989. Interview with Judy Beach, Activities Director, Lucy Corr Nursing Home, Chesterfield, Virginia.

Clark, P. 1988. Journal Entries. Lucy Corr Nursing Home, Chesterfield County, Virginia.

Clark, P., and N. Osgood. 1985. *Seniors on Stage: The Impact of Applied Theatre Techniques on the Elderly*. New York: Praeger Publishers.

Cooney, B. 1982. *Miss Rumphius*. New York: Viking Press.

Corbin, C. 1989. *Strategies 2000: How to Prosper in the New Age*. Austin, Tex.: Eakin Press.

"Danbury School Intergenerational Program." Danbury School, 1700 Danbury Road, Claremont, California, 91711.

Davis, B. 1983. "Drama: A Tool for Nutrition Education with Older Adults." *Journal of Nutrition Education* 15:5.

Dellman-Jenkins, M., D. Lambert, and D. Fruit. 1986. "Old and Young Together: Effect of an Educational Program on Preschoolers' Attitudes Toward Older People." *Childhood Education* 63:206-8, 210-12.

DeRohan, P., ed. 1973. *Federal Theatre Plays*. New York: DeCapo Press.

Drummond, R., et al. 1975. "Project STEP (Seniors Tutor for Educational Progress)." On-Site Validation Report, Easton-Redding Regional School District 9, Connecticut.

Feder, E., and B. Feder. 1981. *The Expressive Arts Therapies: Art, Music, and Dance As Psychotherapy*. New York: Prentice-Hall, Inc.

Firman, J., and A. Stowell. 1980. "Intergenerational School Projects: Examples and Guidelines." *Media and Methods* 17:19,42.

Fleshman, B., and J. L. Fryrear. 1981. *The Arts in Therapy*. Chicago: Nelson Hall.

Freimuth, V., and K. Jamieson. 1979. *Communicating with the Elderly: Shattering Stereotypes*. Urbana, Ill.: ERIC Clearinghouse on Reading and Communication Skills.

"Friendship across the Ages." 1984. Kansas City, Missouri: Camp Fire, Inc.

Gelfand, Donald E. 1982. *Aging: The Ethnic Factor*. Boston: Little, Brown and Company.

Generations United. 1990. Brochure published by Generations United, c/o Child Welfare League of America, Inc., Washington, D.C.

Halpern, James. 1987. *Helping Your Aging Parents*. New York: Fawcett Press.

Handbook For Instruction on Aging. 1978. California State Department of Education, Sacramento.

Hauwiller, J., and Jennings, R. 1981. "Counteracting Age Stereotyping With Young School Children." *Educational Gerontology* 7:183-190.

Hauwiller, J., R. Jennings, and G. Refsland. 1978. *Helping Children Understand Aging Processes: Gerontology in the Elementary Classroom*. Bozeman, Mont.: Montana State University.

Hendricks, G., and K. Hendricks. 1983. *The Moving Center*. Englewood Cliffs, NJ: Prentice Hall.

Heslin, R. 1974. "Steps Toward A Taxomony of Touching." Paper presented at the Midwestern Psychological Association, Chicago.

Hickey, T., L. Hickey, and R. Kalish. 1968. "Children's Perceptions of the Elderly." *The Journal of Genetic Psychology* 112:227-235.

Hillman, H. and K. Abarbanel. 1975. *The Art of Winning Foundation Grants*. New York: Vanguard Press.

Hillman, H., and M. Chamberlain. 1980. *The Art of Winning Corporate Grants*. New York: Vanguard Press.

Hillman, H. and K. Natale. 1977. *The Art of Winning Government Grants*. New York: Vanguard Press.

Hirsch, E. D., Jr. 1987. *Cultural Literacy: What Every American Needs To Know*. Boston: Houghton Mifflin Company.

Ivester, C., and K. King. 1977. "Attitudes of Adolescents toward the Aged." *The Gerontologist* 17:85 - 90.

Jantz, R., C. Seefeldt, A. Galper, and K. Serlock. 1977. "Children's Attitudes Toward the Elderly." *Social Education* 41:518 -23.

John, M. 1977. "Teaching Children about Older Family Members." *Social Education* 41:524-27.

Jones, C. 1986. "Grandparents Read to Special Preschoolers." *Teaching Exceptional Children* 19:36 - 37.

Kearns, D., and D. Doyle. 1988. *Winning the Brain Race*. San Francisco: Institute for Contemporary Studies.

Laban, R., and Lawrence, F.C. 1974. *Effort: Economy In Body Movement*. Boston: Plays, Inc.

Jones, C. 1986. "Grandparents Read to Special Preschoolers." *Teaching Exceptional Children*. 19:36-37.

Justiss, A. 1990. Unpublished request for proposal. Tampa, Florida.

Kearns, D., and D. Doyle. 1988. *Winning the Brain Race*. San Francisco: Institute for Contemporary Studies.

Kebric, R. 1983. "Aging in Pliny's *Letters*: A View from the Second Century A.D." *The Gerontologist* 23:538-45.

Kenny, J. 1988. "Student Community Project in Pittsburgh, Pennsylvania." ACTION, Washington, D.C., VISTA and Student Community Service Programs. Mimeograph.

Kesselman, W. 1980. *Emma*. New York: Harper and Row.

Kirby, Michael. 1976. "Introduction." *The Drama Review* 20:3.

Koste, V. 1978. *Dramatic Play in Childhood: Rehearsal for Life*. New Orleans: Anchorage Press.

Lauzon, L. 1981. "Art Project Spans the Generations." *Design for Arts in Education* 83:41-43.

Lewis-Kane, M., P. McCutcheon, and R. MacDicken. 1986. *Arts Mentor Program: A Manual for Sponsors*. Washington, D.C.: National Council on the Aging.

Lerman, L. and C. Reeverts. 1981. "The Dance Exchange." *Design for Arts in Education* 83:11-20.

Lerman, L. 1984. *Teaching Dance to Senior Adults*. Springfield, IL: Charles D. Thomas Publishers.Lerman, L., and C. Reeverts,. 1981. "The Dance Exchange" *Design for Arts in Education* 83:11-20.

Lubarsky, N. 1987. "A Glance at the Past, a Glimpse of the Future." *Journal of Reading* 30:520-29.

Lyons, C. 1986. "Interagency Alliances Link Young and Old." *Children Today* 15:21-23.

Maclay, E., ed. 1977. *Green Winter: Celebrations of Old Age*. New York: Thomas Y. Crowell Co.

Marx, T. 1983. *Tap Dance: A Beginner's Guide*. Englewood Cliffs, NJ: Prentice Hall.

McCutcheon, P. 1986. *An Arts and Aging Media Sourcebook: Films, Videos, Slide/Tape Shows*. Washington, D.C.: National Council on the Aging.

McCutcheon, P. 1986. *A Manual for Artists: How to Find Work in the Field of Aging*. Washington, D.C.: National Council on the Aging.

McCutcheon, P., and C. Wolf. 1985. *The Resource Guide to People, Places, and Programs in Arts and Aging*. Washington, D.C.: National Council on the Aging.

McGovern, M. 1983. "The Young Keep the Fun in Growing Old." " Activity Director's Guide." 10 Mimeo.

Metal-Corbin, J., D. Corbin, and B. Baker. 1986. "Age Doesn't Matter: Weaving Dance into a Fifth Grade Curriculum." Portions of paper presented at the National AAHPERD Conference in Cincinnati, Ohio, April 13.

Miller, M. 1986. "Elderly Persons as Intergenerational Child Care Providers." *Journal of Employment Counseling* 23:156-61.

Morris, J. 1984. "Project Teen-ager - A Skills Exchange Program: High School Students Volunteering with the Elderly in a Rural Community." Paper presented at the National/International Institute on Social Work in Rural Areas 9th Institute, Orono, Maine, July 28-31.

Naumburg, M. 1977. "Spontaneous Art in Education and Psychotherapy." In *Art Therapy in Theory and Practice*, 2nd ed., edited by E. Ulman and P. Dachinger, 221-22. New York: Shocken Books.

Nelton, S. 1986. "Puppets Promote Understanding." *Nation's Business* 74:70.

Orlock, J., and R. Cornish. 1976. *Short Plays For the Long Living*. Boston: Baker's Plays.

Penrod, J. 1974. *Movement for the Performing Artist*. Palo Alto, CA: Mayfield Publishing Company.

Perschbacher, R. 1984. "An Application of Reminiscence in an Activity Setting: The Tiny Hearts and Aged Hands Program." *The Gerontologist* 24:343-45.

Powell, J., and G. Arquitt. 1978. "Getting the Generations Back Together: A Rationale for Development of Community Based Intergenerational Interaction Programs." *The Family Coordinator* 27:421-26.

Ralston, P., et al. 1986. "Enhancing Intergenerational Contact." Curriculum Guide, Iowa State Department of Public Instruction, Des Moines.

Rice, E. 1959. *The Living Theatre*. New York: Harper and Brothers.

Rogers, C. 1962. "Learning to Be Free," Paper given to a session on "Conformity and Diversity" in the conference on "Man and Civilization," University of California, School of Medicine, San Francisco, 28 January 1962.

Ross, L., and G. Beall. *Intergenerational Programming: Opportunities for National Organizations*. Washington, D.C.: National Council on the Aging.

Russell, J. "Aging in the Public Schools." 1979. *Educational Gerontology: An International Quarterly* 4:19-24.

Seskin, J. 1980. *More than Mere Survival: Conversations with Women over 65*. New York: Newsweek Books.

Short, C. 1971. "The Old One and the Wind." In *Understanding Literature*. 1984. New York: Macmillan.

Smith, C., and Z. Slinkman. 1982. "Generations Together" MF-651. Cooperative Extension Service, Kansas State University, Manhattan, Kansas.

Smith, C., and G. Gutsch. 1985. "Grandletters" MF752, "Program Instructions" MF 752a, "Grandparent Letters" MF 752b, and "Grandchild Letters." Cooperative Extension Service, Kansas State University, Manhattan, March.

Smith, W. 1973. *Granger's Index to Poetry*. Columbia: New York.

Snider, G. 1985. "The Future of Arts Education." excerpted from a paper presented at a panel discussion on "Art and the Universities," Contemporary Art Gallery, Vancouver, B. C., 28 November 1984.

Sohngen, M., and R. Smith. "Images of Old Age in Poetry." 1978. *The Gerontologist* 2:181-86.

Sorgman, M., M. Sorenson, and M. Johnston. 1979. "What Sounds Do I Make When I'm Old?" *Social Education* 43:135-39.

Struntz, K., ed. 1985. *Growing Together: An Intergenerational Sourcebook*. Washington, D.C.: American Association of Retired Persons.

Student papers. 1988. Thomas Dale High School, Chesterfield, Virginia.

Thompson, E. 1979. *On Golden Pond*. New York: Dodd, Mead.

Ventura-Merkel, C. and L. Lidoff. 1983. *Community Planning for Intergenerational Programming*, Volume 8. Washington, D.C.: National Council on the Aging.

Way, Brian. 1967. *Development through Drama*. New York: Humanities Press.

Wertheim, A. 1979. *Radio Comedy*. New York: Oxford University Press.

Williams, Barbara. 1975. *Kevin's Grandma*. New York: E.P. Dutton.

Wilson, C. 1980. *A Treasure Hunt*. Washington, D.C.: U.S. Department of Health, Education, and Welfare, National Institutes of Health, National Institutes of Aging.

"Writing the Living Newspaper." 1937. National Service Bureau of Federal Theatre Project of Works Progress Administration.

"Young and Old Together: A Resource Directory of Intergenerational Programs." 1985. California State Department of Education, Sacramento.

Zahler, D., and K. Zahler. 1988. *Test Your Cultural Literacy*. New York: ARCO.

Index

About the Author

PATCH CLARK teaches English and Theatre at Thomas Dale High School in Virginia and is an adjunct faculty member at John Tyler Community College. She teaches a course in theatre and language arts at Lucy Corr Nursing Home in association with the college and is the co-author of *Seniors on Stage* (Praeger, 1985).